Acid Reflux Diet

The Complete Guide to Cook Healthy Food for Healing and Prevent GERD, LPR, and Acid Reflux Disease with Quick & Easy Meal Plans and delicious Recipes including Vegan and Gluten-Free

Sable Delight

ACID REFLUX DIET

To Giuseppe

TABLE OF CONTENTS

Thanks Mum

DESCRIPTION

If you have ever felt heartburn, usually described as "fire in the chest," then you will know how uncomfortable this condition can be. It usually occurs after eating heavy and fatty food, smoking a lot, or drinking alcohol. This problem is more common than you think. Around 3 billion people in the world suffer from this condition at least once a day.

Modern lifestyles, full of stress, poor diets, and poor eating habits, with unhealthy and processed foods, lots of caffeine, alcohol, and carbonated drinks, have a harmful effect on our digestive tract and whole body.

In medical terms, acidity can be described as acid indigestion. This burning sensation in the chest and/or upper abdomen appears due to the regurgitation of gastric acid to the esophagus. Unlike the stomach, which is covered by protective cells, our esophagus does not have this protection. Naturally, when stomach acids and digestive juices return, they cause serious inflammation and damage inside the esophagus.

Preventing heartburn should be your number one priority to keep your digestive tract normal and healthy. The best way to do this is to change your daily eating habits. The most common acidity triggers are:

- Alcohol
- Caffeine
- Free medications
- Carbonated drinks
- Acid foods and juices
- Smoking

These irritants increase the production of acid in the stomach and should be avoided. However, there is much more you can do to cure the damage caused by years and even decades of bad eating habits.

This book will help you understand what causes acid reflux and how you can take care of it.

INTRODUCTION

Congratulations on purchasing *Acid Reflux Diet,* and thank you for doing so.

There are plenty of books on this subject on the market, thanks again for choosing this one! Every effort was made to ensure it is full of as much useful information as possible. Please enjoy!

Since we became professional nutritionists, our views on nutrition, health, and the very attitude to life have radically changed. We both feel younger for a dozen years, and we are often given compliments about our appearance. Throughout the day, we feel a surge of energy, are in a good mood, and have completely forgotten about fatigue. And we are not at all averse to skipping a glass—another wine or enjoying a chocolate dessert—excellent health allows us some excesses without little serious consequences.

If you are interested in their own health and proper nutrition, then this guide for a summary of best practices, based on the latest achievements of science. The first part is devoted to food products and their impact on your mood and well-being; the second part you will learn, what diet to choose to deal with those or other illnesses, how to maintain a healthy weight and fight allergies. In addition, we introduce you to different ways of cooking, as well as give delicious recipes, which will help you maintain a healthy lifestyle. We are confident that our book will help you understand how proper nutrition is important for physical and spiritual health.

Thanks again for choosing this book and make sure to leave a short review on Amazon if you enjoy it, I'd really love to hear your thoughts!

CHAPTER 1:

YOUR LIFESTYLE

As specialists—nutritionists, people constantly turn to us with complaints about various kinds of ailments, the reasons for which are far from obvious. Some diseases can be treated with conventional medicine, but in many cases, the true cause of the disease drugs persists, and in order to figure it out, you need to know which way is the patient.

Below is a list of the 20 most common complaints that our patients come to us with. If in this list, you find something that you are concerned about and after reading the relevant paragraph, you answer "yes" to most of the questions, note the possible causes. For example, a feeling of constant fatigue can be caused by stress. However, the simultaneous presence of a high need for sugar and caffeine can also indicate a tendency to allergies or a violation of the normal composition of the intestinal microflora. A common denominator for many symptoms is the intestinal condition and efficiency, which in turn, is closely interconnected with the liver and pancreas. Normalization of the digestive system leads to the fact that it is possible to get rid of unwanted symptoms relatively quickly. You can learn more about various diseases in the subsequent sections of the book. Keep in mind, however, that the causes of the disease listed here are not always the only ones and our recommendations in no way replace the advice of a doctor.

Fatigue/Tiredness

- Do you feel constant tiredness?
- Are you irritable and quick-tempered?
- You do not feel rested after sleep?
- Do you feel overwhelmed during the day?
- Do you often feel "out of place" for no apparent reason?
- Do you consume a lot of sugar, tea, and coffee?

Possible causes: violation of intestinal patency and food allergy, violation of the normal composition of the intestinal microflora and fungal infection of the intestine, exposure to toxic metals, low blood pressure, low thyroid function, lack of carbohydrates and fluctuations in blood sugar, lack of certain nutrients.

Pain and Inflammation

- Do you feel pain in the joints or fingers? Do your joints swell?
- Do you often have pain in your neck, shoulders, or back?
- The foundation of your diet consists of foods "fast food"?
- Do you take painkillers daily, such as ibuprofen?

Possible causes: poor digestibility of food, violation of the intestinal microflora composition and fungal infection of the intestine, lack of polyunsaturated fatty acids (PUFAs), autoimmune disease, thyroid dysfunction, trauma, impaired hepatic detoxification.

Indigestion (Dyspepsia)

- Do you often experience stomach pain after eating? Do you often have constipation?

- Are there leftovers from undigested food in your stool? Does burping bother you?
- Do you abuse chewing gum?

Possible causes: decreased acidity of the stomach, lack of digestive enzymes, bacterial infection or parasitic invasion, poor digestibility of food, stomach or duodenal ulcer, and frequent use of antacids, impaired liver function.

Meteorism and Intestinal Bloating

- Do you feel bloating immediately after eating? Do you often have flatulence?
- Do you often have intestinal colic? Do you abuse alcohol?
- Do you have a craving for sweets, bread, pasta, wine?

Possible causes: decreased acidity of the stomach, lack of digestive enzymes, bacterial/parasitic infection, poor digestibility, impaired intestinal motility, poor diet.

Headaches and Migraines

- Do you often resort to painkillers, to remove a headache?
- Do you eat a lot of cheese, chocolate, and dairy products?
- Do headaches and migraines worsen during menstruation?
- Do you have a food allergy?
- Do you have digestive problems?

Possible causes: poor digestibility of food, a violation of intestinal patency, exposure to toxic metals, narrowing the lumen of blood vessels—due to smoking, alcohol abuse, lack of supervision over blood sugar, or injury, impaired vision.

PMS (Premenstrual Syndrome)

- Do you have a malfunction in your regularity?
- Are you drawn to chocolate before your period?
- Are you irritable, quick-tempered, or have increased excitement before menstruation?
- Do you notice a monthly weight gain, water retention?
- Do you experience premenstrual cramps?

Possible causes: lack of magnesium and vitamin B 6, circulatory disturbance, hormonal imbalance, disturbance in the level of the pituitary hormone, stress.

Excitation and Nervousness

- Are you prone to pessimism?
- Do you have a lot of filled teeth?
- Have you lived in an industrial area since childhood?
- Are you craving sugar and sweets?
- Do you drink coffee and soft drinks daily?

Possible causes: exposure to substances, pollutants, environment, and toxic metals, a violation of the composition of the chemical elements of the brain, an imbalance of amino acids, impaired liver function, poor digestibility of food, fungal infection, stress.

Depression

- Do you eat irregularly?
- Does food help you get rid of a bad mood?
- Do you lack motivation in life?
- Do you suffer from insomnia?

Possible causes: impaired blood sugar, exposure to substances, environmental pollutants, and toxic metals, a violation of the chemical composition of the brain cells, disruption of the normal composition of intestinal microflora, a fungal infection, poor assimilation of food, stress, hereditary diseases, the abuse of stimulants.

High Arterial Pressure or High Level of Cholesterol; Pains for the Breast

- Do you have a strong heartbeat?
- Do you have shortness of breath after climbing stairs?
- Do you have tingling sensations in your limbs?
- Do you add salt to food during its preparation, as well as to ready-made meals?
- Do you smoke?
- Is fried food the bulk of your diet?
- Does your weight exceed the ideal weight by more than 10 kilograms?

Possible causes: sedentary lifestyle, unbalanced diet, diet, rich in saturated fats and fried foods, decreased thyroid function, increased adrenaline rush by the adrenal glands, smoking, increased alcohol consumption, increased salt intake, heart disease.

Diabetes (Type II—Insulin Independent)

- Do you often eat sweets?
- Do you experience mood swings throughout the day?
- Do you often behave illogically, enter into disputes?
- Are you often thirsty?
- Do you often feel the urge to urinate?
- Do you constantly feel tired?

Possible causes: pancreatic insufficiency (decreased insulin production), a diet high in carbohydrates, a lack of digestive enzymes, obesity, a sedentary lifestyle, impaired liver function, increased adrenaline, a lack of chromium and vitamin B 3.

Infertility (Male and Female)

- Have you unsuccessfully tried to conceive a child for one year and more?
- Do you regularly drink alcohol?
- Are you under fatigue?
- Does your diet include 'fast food' as a major part of your diet?
- Do you live in an area with a high level of environmental pollution?

Possible causes: hormonal imbalance, bacterial or parasitic infection, exposure to toxic metals and substances, polluting the environment, shortage of certain nutrients and substances (polyunsaturated fatty acids, magnesium, zinc, certain amino acids), poor digestibility of food, anatomical reasons.

Allergy

- Do you suffer from hay fever or rhinitis (runny nose)?
- Do you often have headaches?
- Do you experience palpitations after eating? Do you have skin rashes?
- Do you have a craving for certain products for nutrition?
- Do you often have depression?

Possible causes: disturbance of normal microflora and patency of the intestines, vaccinations, environmental pollution, decreased liver function, imbalance in polyunsaturated fatty acids, increased adrenaline rush by the adrenal glands, decreased acidity of the stomach, lack of digestive enzymes.

Skin Diseases

- Have you recently returned from a long trip?
- Does your skin suffer from heat and direct sunlight?
- Do you tend to be under the influence of stress for a long time?
- Do you regularly drink alcohol?
- Do dairy and instant foods make up a significant proportion of your diet?
- Do you use constantly in your daily diet which—or certain foods?

Possible causes: poor assimilation of food (especially dairy and wheat products, as well as citrus fruits), hormonal changes, parasitic invasion, lack of polyunsaturated fatty acids, lack of vitamin C, indiscriminate nutrition.

Eczema and Asthma

- Do you have a lot of fried foods and meat in your diet?
- Do you eat dairy products daily?
- Do you drink alcohol regularly?
- Do you regularly use medications?

Possible causes: poor digestibility of food (in particular, dairy and wheat products, as well as citrus fruits), an imbalance of polyunsaturated fatty acids, poor posture, allergies to cosmetics and cleansers, diet, rich in saturated fats.

Excessive Activity

- Do you eat a lot of sweets?
- Is the basis of your diet "fast food"?
- Do you drink soft and fizzy drinks, containing dyes?
- Are you already taking drugs for excessive activity?
- Do you regularly take aspirin?

Possible reasons: food allergy and poor digestibility of food, hypersensitivity to food additives, sensitivity to salicylates (aspirin-like substances, which are added to certain food products), lack of polyunsaturated fatty acids, exposure to substances, polluting and toxic metals, vaccinations.

Diarrhea/Constipation

- Do you suffer from bouts of diarrhea, alternating with constipation?
- Are fruits and vegetables rare guests at your table?
- Do you rarely exercise?

- Do you use standard painkillers?
- Do you take a laxative?

Possible causes: inflammation and decreased intestinal motility, lack of fiber in food, sedentary lifestyle, bacterial/parasitic infection, poor posture, smoking, alcohol abuse, impaired liver function.

Cold, Influenza, Frequent Infections

- Have you recently lost a loved one?
- Have you recently had surgery?
- Are you often stressed?
- Do you eat a lot of dairy products?
- Do you suffer from food or other allergies?

Possible causes: decreased immunity, increased release of adrenaline by the adrenal glands, the inflammatory process and reduced intestinal motility, bacterial infections, lack of vitamins A, C, E, zinc, and selenium.

Fungal Infections and Cystitis

- Do you have problems with digestion?
- Do you often eat animal products?
- Is there a lot of sugar in your diet?
- Do you have mouth sores?
- Do you have frequent urination?

Possible causes: disturbance of normal microflora and intestinal motility, bacterial infections, diet high acidity.

Nutrition and Obesity

- Are you afraid to eat?
- Do you constantly think about food?
- Do you experience a craving for food of a certain kind?
- Are you used to weigh yourself daily?
- Is your weight more than normal by more than 20 kg?
- Do you try to keep your gastronomic habits secret?

Possible causes: thyroid dysfunction, lack of amino acids, lack of zinc and vitamin B 6, chromium, and vitamin B 3, inactive or excessively mobile lifestyle, pancreatic insufficiency, impaired blood sugar.

Loss of Attention/Memory

- Do you eat irregularly?
- Do you have a lot of teeth in your mouth which are sealed with amalgam fillings?
- Do you regularly consume beverages, contain caffeine?
- Do you feel a craving for food of a certain kind?
- Do you suffer from any digestive disorders?

Possible causes: toxic effects of metals and products, environmental pollution, bacterial and parasitic infections, impaired blood sugar, lack of many nutrients.

CHAPTER 2:

HOW TO CONTROL WEIGHT

Many people understand that it is time to change the diet, but they only realize that they need to get rid of excess weight. If you are aiming to do the same and you, we will give you the same advice that our customers: you lose weight when you go on a healthy diet. Place order to lead a healthy life, and you become more aware, which means eating right, and why you are gaining weight.

The food industry is largely subject to vorotilam—the world of cosmetics and fashion, which tell us how we should look, to feel healthy. Fabulous money is spent on advertising weight loss products and diet drinks. Although diets really help some people, in general, in our opinion, to go on a diet is completely unjustified. We both had to deal with the clients, who have experienced serious health problems, but nevertheless refused to pass the health food just because, that it consisted of products, from which "you can put on weight." Such clients preferred to be sick even further, if only not to gain a couple of extra pounds.

Why Diets Do Not Help

Rarely given week, anyone—do not try to offer us another elaborate diet, designed once and for all solve our overweight problem. Events each time develop according to the same scenario: in the first days, a person really loses weight, but this is explained solely by the loss of moisture, not fat. The outcome is always disappointing.

We had to deal with clients, who sat on a diet is not safe, and ultimately undermine their own health. For example, diet, enriched advantageously protein food, can lead to a softening of the bones and kidneys diseases over time; a low-fat diet can disrupt the activity of the endocrine glands and the brain, which will inevitably affect the human psyche.

Is it Realistic to Lose Five Pounds in Five Days?

The key to the safe and effective management of its own weight is to understand what the body loses during weight loss. When dieting, we consume less food (and fewer calories). This causes that the body, forced to resort to its reserves, begins to consume glycogen, used as an energy reserve. Glycogen, which is deposited in the liver and muscles, is soluble. Therefore, the weight loss that is observed in the first days after starting any such diet simply reflects the loss of water. This is what you promise unscrupulous advertisers, that promise, that in five days, you dropped five pounds. Therefore, since you are losing weight due not to fat, but to liquid, the effect of losing weight is purely speculative. If you follow the recommendations of such a diet for a long time, the body gets used to consuming less food and accustomed to extract the right amount of energy from an impoverished diet. This explains the effect of the "plateau", well familiar to fans of restrictive diets, which, to his chagrin, discovered that in spite of the half-starved life, they do not shed more weight.

Erratic Diets – Thyroid Dysfunction

There are people who randomly jump from one diet to another. They lock themselves in a vicious circle: first they lose weight, then they gain weight, they lose it again, and then, and inevitably, they grow even stronger. Disappointment—for this is so great, that these people often develop depression, reduced self-esteem, and even hormonal balance is disturbed.

The speed, with which our body burns food and converts it into energy (metabolic rate) is controlled by the thyroid gland, situated at the base of the neck. This gland is necessary for energy production, and it determines our daily well-being. People who follow different diets disturb the delicate balance of hormones as it enters the thyroid gland and produced by it, with the result that the metabolic rate drops. In turn, this leads to a slowdown in thyroid function and restoration of the level of stored glycogen; all this makes weight loss an unattainable dream.

Stress

When stress produced by two hormones: cortisone and DHEA (see. P.58). Stress leads to a change in hormonal balance and can contribute to the formation of fats, even with a limited amount of food consumed. In this case, a man, sitting on a diet, do not lose weight, why diet itself becomes for him an additional stress factor.

Allergies and Intolerances

Sometimes it happens that our body develops intolerance to a particular kind of food every day. When such occurs, the body itself retains the liquid to protect the most sensitive organs, e.g., the gastrointestinal tract. Water retention in tissues leads to swelling and weight gain.

Intolerance to wheat products, a whole cup of cereal with toast in the morning, a sandwich with salad for the day, and pasta with ketchup for evening. We have shown that the exclusion of wheat from the diet leads to increased metabolism and weight loss rate. If you suspect yourself of food intolerance, keep a food diary—with it, you will determine the frequency of consumption of the same foods.

Blood Sugar Disorder

We found that almost all people, vainly trying to lose weight, impaired blood sugar. Normalization of hormonal imbalance is the first step to that, to lose weight. It also helps to reduce the inflammatory response, improve mood, increase energy levels, as well as eliminate the constant feeling of hunger.

There is nothing healthier than fresh and juicy fruits and vegetables. The nutrients they contain support the function of the thyroid gland and the optimal metabolic rate, and the high fiber content helps to remove excess fat from the body. It is most useful to eat raw fruits and vegetables, as cooking leads to the destruction of nutrients and vitamins.

Surprisingly, the fact is that we need fats to maintain a normal weight. Unsaturated fatty acids, which are contained in the nuts, oily fish, seeds, and olive oil, are essential for removing fat from the fat tissues and for weight regulation. All cells in our body contain a fat (lipid) membrane, which protects them from possible damage, passes nutrients into the cell and helps to remove toxins and toxins. This lipid membrane consists of unsaturated fatty acids, which are not produced by the body and, therefore, must come from food. The lack of unsaturated fatty acids leads to increased rigidity of cell membranes, as a result of which toxins and fats are not removed from the cells. Fats are condensed, and getting rid of them over time becomes harder and harder. That's why to get rid of fat and cellulite is necessary to consume food containing unsaturated fatty acids. Most of them are found in fatty fish: sardines, mackerel, herring, tuna, and salmon. For vegetarians, flaxseed, pumpkin, sunflower and sesame seeds are a great source of unsaturated fatty acids. You can also consume olive oil in moderation.

Make the right choice—a great menu for every day Forget your prejudices, look at the below table, and make sure, that the typical daily diet cannot only be balanced but also varied and delightfully delicious!

Breakfast

A glass of fresh vegetable or fruit juice, as well as one of the following:

- tofu
- millet porridge
- natural bio-yogurt with any fruit, as well as ground pumpkin, sesame, or sunflower seeds.
- corn flakes without sugar or granola * (* a mixture of flattened oats with additives of brown sugar, raisins, coconuts, and nuts—for making breakfast cereals—hereinafter approx. transl.) with rice milk.
- omelet with tomatoes or mushrooms

Lunch

One of the following options to choose from:

- apple or pear with cottage cheese
- a handful of pumpkin seeds, almonds, or walnuts
- half avocado
- Cornflakes without sugar, with hummus*

*Paste made from Turkey peas with sesame seeds.

Dinner

Vegetable soup with a green salad, as well as any four raw vegetables from this list: broccoli, chopped cabbage, grated carrots or pumpkin, beets, mushrooms, green onions, radishes, cauliflower, peas, sweet corn

And also, some of this:

- homemade cheese piece of chicken breast (skinless)
- jar of canned tuna, sardines, or salmon
- grilled fish with stewed vegetables

Plus:

- fruits, for example, banana, apple, some berries, canned cherries (without syrup or sugar)

In addition to diet, it is very useful to exercise regularly, which helps maintain normal blood sugar levels. Of course, with a tendency to a sedentary lifestyle, you have to force yourself. It's not easy to do physical training intensively. Nevertheless, if some people achieve the desired goal by visiting the gym, others are satisfied with daily walks, or, for example, go to work three times a week. Do not hesitate—make a decision today and start exercising regularly. For weight loss, a daily massage of the entire surface of the body is also useful, with the help of which the outflow of lymph increases, the reserves of body fat burn faster. For massage, use better not with a synthetic product, but with a brush made of natural bristles, massaging the skin with wide movements towards the center of the body.

Surprisingly, the fact is that we need fats to maintain a normal weight. Especially useful are unsaturated fatty acids, which help to remove stored fat from adipose tissue.

Table of healthy food, below, is an example, how to choose a diet to control blood sugar levels, increase vitality, and improve health, against the background of maintaining a healthy weight. At every meal, follow the principle of combining a certain amount of protein and carbohydrates to maintain normal blood sugar levels and rid yourself of the constant and obsessive desire to eat.

High Tea

Select some of these:

- a piece of fruit (such as an orange)
- a small tassel of grapes or plums
- a handful of nuts and seeds
- a couple of oatmeal cakes with avocado gravy

Supper Serving a protein dish, for example:

- fish, turkey, or chicken with a side dish of three (at least) vegetables and brown or Canadian rice.
- rice or noodle with stewed chicken
- tofu with a side dish of stewed vegetables, including red pepper, carrots, beans, ginger, onions, and mushrooms

Snack at Bedtime

Select some of these:

- homemade cheese and two banana oatmeal cakes
- rice pudding with hummus or peanut butter (without salt and sugar).

CHAPTER 3:

FOOD ALLERGY

Food allergies are a fairly common disease. Allergies today are much more common than half a century ago. This may be due to environmental pollution, the use of pesticides, as well as an abundance of other chemicals, which we use or which we face in everyday life. It is estimated that every year, we are exposed to about 3 thousand different chemicals—so that an increase in the number of allergic diseases is not surprising.

Our immune system is daily exposed to chemicals, which we get from food and drinks, as well as potentially toxic molecules, which we breathe. This constant battle leads to liver overload and, as a result, to an increase in allergic reactions.

In Britain, the most common food allergens are wheat, dairy products, citrus fruits, and chicken eggs. In the process of human evolution, wheat products appeared relatively recently. People started cultivating wheat only about ten thousand years ago. While it is not clear, it reflects low tolerability of products, comprising wheat, poor adaptability to the human body wheat, or blame pesticides, herbicides, and other possible toxic impurities. Wheat products often make up a significant proportion of the consumer diet in the West, which also explains the high prevalence of food allergies there.

The most dangerous form of allergies to cereal products is gluten allergy, which is caused by oats, wheat, rye, and barley. Users, subject to such diseases like celiac disease, cannot tolerate these cereals in any form. In the most acute cases, gluten allergy can be life-threatening since gluten causes erosion of the internal walls of the digestive tract and prevents the absorption of essential nutrients.

What is Called an Allergy, and What is Not?

There is a certain mixture of the concepts of allergy and intolerance. If their manifestations are similar to each other, then the reasons are completely different. Allergies, in general, are defined as an immediate response to any stimulus, in response to which the immune system produces antibodies against the molecules—offenders.

Intolerance means a delayed reaction to food (often it develops only after a few days), which manifests itself in the form of a wide variety of symptoms, at first glance, not even related.

Moreover, many symptoms are generally difficult to directly relate to food intolerance. They are so diverse that they are often confused with manifestations of completely different diseases.

Similar symptoms include depression, joint pain, under-eye swelling, yellowing, paleness and/or dry skin, "haze" (difficulty concentrating and decreased mental clarity), shortness of breath, constipation and/or diarrhea, mouth sores ("cold on the lips"), runny nose, indigestion, rash, bags and/or shadows under the eyes, bedwetting in children.

Do You Have Any Allergies or Intolerances?

There are certain differences between food allergies and food intolerances. Diagnosis helps the reaction of the organism in response to the food, causing suspicion.

Allergy Intolerance manifestation of a reaction immediately with a delay causes histamine and antibodies, symptoms like urticaria, rash, itching, rapid pulse, swelling, vomiting, fatigue, swelling, trembling, blush, muscle pain, dark circles sudden fatigue under the eyes, headaches, and migraines.

Genetic Factor

Although quite often, children with allergies inherit the disease from their parents, allergy is inherited is not always. It was found that the children of parents suffering from asthma, eczema, or hay fever (atopic allergy) themselves have a heightened sensitivity, in particular, if these allergic diseases are manifested in both parents. The genes that determine the suppression of the formation of IgE, immunoglobulins, which are mediators of the acute inflammatory reaction to specific allergens, are guilty of this. However, genes are not the only reason for allergies. For example, genetically identical twins do not necessarily develop allergic reactions in response to the same allergens. This proves that in the event of allergies play a role, and other factors, for example, environmental factors, bacterial and viral infections, stress, and so on.

Digestion and Allergy

Two-thirds of the components constituting the body's immune system, located in the digestive tract, which explains the high sensitivity of the digestive system to food and other allergens. Very big troubles arise with increased reproduction in the intestines of Candida albicans fungi.

Useful Advice

If for lunch you prefer to eat sandwiches, then, in order to avoid the development of food intolerance, try to diversify them every day. Eat black, white, or gray bread with chicken, tuna, cheese, or salad.

Although Candida fungi live in the intestines and are normal, when the immune system is suppressed, they can begin to multiply intensely. At the same time, they cause ulceration of the mucous membranes and intestinal walls, as a result of which food particles penetrate into the formed holes and provoke an exacerbation of immune reactions. Candidiasis is often the cause of headaches and migraines associated with food intolerance.

How to Deal with Allergies and Food Intolerances

With normal digestion and a healthy immune system, problems with allergies and food intolerance do not occur. At the first stage of the fight against these ailments, it is necessary to identify the source of irritation. To do this, consult a professional nutritionist.

In children, manifestation of typical symptoms often can be quickly removed, eliminating them from the food, which causes these reactions. For example, the symptoms of overactive or restlessness, associated with a decrease in attention, usually is enough to exclude the child from the diet products, containing artificial additives or food dyes.

Dietitian consultations also help to solve many long-standing health problems in adults. Often eat seasonal products, daily Diversify your diet, and you'll soon get rid of many of the problems caused by food intolerance.

Allergy Tests

Many types of products are irritants not only for the digestive system but also for the whole organism. Uses a variety of types of assays to detect allergic reactions of a simple skin test to comprehensive blood analysis when determining the level of antibodies in response to a variety of foods. The results of these tests do not always allow us to make a final conclusion because there are both false-positive and false-negative results. Upon further examination, it often turns out that the patient has certain disorders of digestion, which is responsible for this type of intolerance. To help you figure it out, we will discuss below, what is a healthy digestive system, and give recommendations on how to keep it in optimal condition. With the help of the measures, you will overcome the unpleasant consequences, associated with food intolerance, and can again enjoy your favorite food.

Food Diaries

From my own experience, we know that using a food diary, in which you regularly write not only what you eat or drink but also the subsequent reactions of the organism, is useful for identifying those products, which are associated with these reactions. It is advisable to record not only physical but also emotional reactions. For example, some people say that during the day after taking the tomatoes, they start to hurt the joints. There are edema and increased irritability; in other patients, taking bread or pasta can cause depression, headache, or even sneezing.

Food Allergy

However, at the slightest suspicion on food intolerance, it is desirable to get your food diary acquainted with an expert dietician. If your body is characterized by delayed reactions, determining the true cause of intolerance can be quite difficult.

Anaphylactic Shock

Anaphylactic shock is an extremely acute, dangerous, and often life-threatening reaction to an antigenic stimulus. Anaphylactic shock can cause peanuts, due to which the labels of some products have warned that they contain peanuts or other nuts, which can cause allergic reactions in sensitive individuals. Sometimes such reactions cause mollusks; however, on the product packaging containing them, you will not find decals. Anaphylactic shock can also be stung by bees and wasps. For symptoms of anaphylactic shock, you should immediately take the victim to the hospital, as he may need an injection of adrenaline (epinephrine). Some people who are susceptible to this disease constantly carry these medications with them, and then, perhaps, you will do the injection yourself. With severe swelling and difficulty breathing, the patient needs to insert a straw in his mouth.

Complete Food Immunity

Sometimes there are people who cannot tolerate "literally anything". As a rule, this is due to severe intestinal dysbiosis, in which the intestines are so inflamed, that food particles directly from the intestines enter the bloodstream. In such cases, it is necessary to carry out targeted treatment to get rid of the inflammation.

It also happens that the liver cannot withstand overload associated with prolonged use of high doses of alcohol, sugar, or drugs. When the liver is "podsazheny", it exhibits many symptoms, typical for food intolerance. In such cases, the nutritionist should advise you on a diet that helps restore liver function.

In some people, prone to allergies, immediately after a meal may develop a dangerous reaction, which, in the absence of proper and prompt treatment, can even be life-threatening. These reactions occur within a few minutes after eating, and you can recognize them by the following symptoms.

Cooking is not only an art but also a pleasure. If food is cooked quality, she and tastier, and looks attractive. However, heat treatment of products often leads to a decrease in their nutritional value. Although we recommend eating as much raw food as you can (if it is not injurious to health), we are aware that it is not suitable for everyone. It follows that it is necessary to find a middle ground between taste and nutritional value.

Culinary processing changes the structure of food products, contributing to their translation in a better digestible form. However, in some cases, a culinary treatment can change the properties of the product is so, it is a potential carcinogen. For example, in oils, overcooked chemical structure is disrupted, causing them to become harmful, in particular, for the cardiovascular system.

Some cooking and cooking methods preserve the nutritional value and water content of foods better than others. Vitamin C and all B vitamins are water-soluble and are easily destroyed by intensive heat treatment.

Steam Processing

Steaming is one of the most effective ways to preserve nutrients. Bring a small volume of water to a boil and place food (usually vegetables or fish) in a double boiler over boiling water. Just a few minutes later, the food will be ready. Dense vegetables, such as carrots and broccoli, are steamed for about five minutes, while a minute is enough to cook spinach. After steam processing, vegetables retain their shape, color, fiber structure and do not lose nutritional value.

Missing ten minutes to prepare the steam fish, and such a method allows you to save not only the "good" fats, which is famous for the fish but the water-soluble B vitamins. Fish can be steamed over boiling water, in which ginger, lemon juice, or aromatic herbs are added—this is an excellent way to improve its taste.

Boiled Food

Cooking, especially vegetables, by cooking is the best way to deprive it not only of attractiveness but also of the lion's share of nutrients. If carrots are boiled for more than ten minutes, most of the vitamin C goes into water. Well, then it would be more useful to drink this water and throw the carrots!

Remember: when cooking vegetables destroyed about 40% of the B vitamins and 70% of vitamin C. The more water in the pan, the greater the loss of vitamins. The situation still is aggravated if the vegetables are cut into small pieces since the contact surface with water, and in this case, the thermal factor increases, and this leads to further loss of nutrients.

Cooking Methods

In many countries, when cooking vegetables in water, it is customary to add salt. This is completely useless: the diet of most people is already oversaturated with salt. Salt not only violates the balance of sodium and water in the body but also—the normal rhythm of the heart muscle. All fruits and vegetables already contain sodium, and only taste buds, dulled by excessive consumption of alcohol and sugar, need additional salt. So, if you already cook food, then try to do it faster and use as little water as possible. It is more useful to cook food for a couple.

How deep and shallow roasting enhances the taste and appearance of food, but the resulting product is fraught with the potential for harm.

Fried Food

How deep and superficial roasting improves the taste and appearance of food, but the resulting product is fraught with the potential for harm. Despite the fact that the process of cooking takes little time, excessive heat destroys nutrients and damage the heat-sensitive lipids contained, for example, in fatty fish and poultry. Cooking oil, used for frying, have so-called "point fuming": temperature, at which the oil is combusted. Each type of oil has its own "smoke point"—at the highest temperature, olive oil "extra-virgin" burns.

When frying food, many free radicals are formed. The so-called atoms have a damaging effect on the body—they contribute to the development of cancer, cardiovascular disease ("Arteriosclerosis and atherosclerosis"), and premature aging. The harmful effect of free radicals can be counteracted by consuming food, rich in antioxidants ("Splendid five"). However, antioxidants are easily damaged when exposed to high temperatures, characteristic of the cooking process. Refried or even a little—a little burnt food is potentially carcinogenic. Even the smoke from frying food can be dangerous—the cook, who often cook fried dishes, a higher risk of developing lung cancer or cancer of the larynx, than their counterparts.

Both water-soluble (B and C) and fat-soluble (D, A, K, and E) vitamins are lost in both types of frying. For example, when frying meat or chicken, the content of B vitamins is reduced by 30%.

Stir-Frying

Although roasting food while stirring in a wok * (*A deep-frying pan with two ear-shaped handles, commonly used in Chinese cuisine) is considered a healthier way of cooking compared to deep frying, nevertheless, it is also frying. If it is possible as the loss of nutrients and chemical modification of fats.

However, oil is consumed much less with this method, and the cooking process, thanks to the even distribution of heat in the wok, is also significantly accelerated. In addition, constant mixing can significantly reduce harm.

When the oil in the wok warms up, add one tablespoon of water and one tablespoon of soy sauce to it. Thanks to this, the oil will not burn out, and the resulting steam will contribute to better cooking. Better yet, pre-process the food a bit, and then "bring" it to the desired condition in the wok.

Microwave Cooking

With this cooking method, the required temperature is created by water molecules contained in the products, which begin to move under the influence of radiation. Waves bounce off the walls of the oven and penetrate the food. The nutritional properties of vegetables remain very high, which is one of the advantages of this method. And yet, for their better preservation, it is preferable to cook steamed vegetables.

One of the main problems encountered with this method of cooking is the selection of products. The so-called "prepared meals" designed for microwave cooking contain substances harmful to the body's sugar, salt, and often—hydrogenated fats. In addition, under the influence of microwave radiation, these substances are more susceptible to certain molecular changes as a result of which free radicals harmful to health can form.

Stews and Soups

Extinguishing cooking requires prolonged simmering. With stews, as well as casseroles and soups along with cooked foods we consume and the liquid, in which the food is prepared, as it contains valuable nutrients, have fallen into the water.

The advantage of stews is slow cooking at temperatures below the boiling point. It follows from this that the process of destruction of vitamins and inorganic substances, which accelerates with increasing temperature, is much slower. In addition, protein products are better absorbed, since when quenched, the fibers degenerate and are easier to digest.

Some fruits in the process of stewing even acquire useful properties. For example, in prunes with this cooking method, enzymes are released. In stewed fruits, the naturally sweet taste increases, so it is better to consume them with a small amount of unsweetened bio-yogurt.

Roasting

The preparation of meat, poultry, and vegetables in various ovens and roasters is widely used in Western countries and has not lost popularity so far. At the same time, if the oven is not too overheated, the fat content in the product remains at the initial level. However, burning fats acquire potential carcinogenic properties. Browning formed, mainly due to carbohydrates, undergo changes due to the high temperature.

When baking food in the oven, there is an inevitable loss of some water-soluble vitamins, in particular, vitamin C and B complex. As a rule, the content of vitamins B is reduced by 25%; however, with increasing temperature, the process of destruction of vitamins is exacerbated.

Grill

In summer, many people like to grill kebabs or cook on a metal grill over coals. Usually, meat and fish are fried in this way. Most people prefer a bit of undercooked food in this. However, it will be recalled, that burnt food potentially carcinogenic—in direct contact with the walls of the throat and the digestive tract can be damaged cells, resulting in accumulation of free radicals.

To reduce the harm of food, cooked on the grill, try to coal temperature was as high as possible. They should be red-hot, but in no case—do not burn. On direct fire, especially using different kiln, roast meat can—with a crust—form a variety of chemicals and a health hazard.

Raw Food

The raw food content of useful nutrients as possible. Of course, we do not offer you to eat raw meat or gnaw grains of cereals, but fresh vegetables, fruits, nuts, and seeds must be eaten every day. Raw foods contain their own digestive enzymes, which reduces the load on the pancreas. Raw foods are high in fiber, which helps to remove toxins and excess cholesterol from the body.

If you are used to eating "finished foods", we urge you to spare no time and pay more attention to healthy eating.

Useful Advice

Soaking food, intended for cooking on a grill, in olive oil (rich in vitamin E) bit protects against the damaging effects of free radicals generated.

CHAPTER 4:

ENERGY AND EMOTIONS: GOOD NUTRITION, GOOD MOOD

From the food we consume, energy is produced, which is necessary to carry out any functions of our body—from the distance and the ability to speak to the digestion and breathing. But why do we often complain about lack of energy, irritability, or lethargy? The answer is, what kind of food is our daily diet.

Energy Production

In addition to air and water, our body constantly needs a regular inflow of food, which provides energy and supplies required for movement, breathing, thermoregulation, heart function, blood flow, and brain activity. It is amazing, but even resting our brain consumes about 50% of energy, stored by absorbed from food, and energy consumption increases dramatically during intense brain activity, for example, during exams. How is the conversion of food into energy?

During digestion, described in more detail in the corresponding section, food breaks down into individual glucose molecules, which then enter the bloodstream through the intestinal wall.

With blood flow, glucose is transferred to the liver, where it is filtered and stored in reserve. Pituitary (located in the brain, endocrine gland) takes the pancreas and thyroid hormones signal emission, which causes the liver to throw the accumulated glucose into the bloodstream, whereupon blood delivers it to the organs and muscles, which need it.

Having reached the desired organ, glucose molecules penetrate into the cells, where they are converted into a source of energy, which is available for use by cells. Thus, the process of constant supply of organs with energy depends on the level of glucose in the blood.

In order to increase the body's energy reserves, we have to use certain kinds of products, in particular, can increase the metabolic rate and maintain the required level of energy. To understand how all this happens, consider the following questions:

How Does Food Turn into Energy?

There are mitochondria in every cell in our body. Here, components, included in the food products, undergo a series of chemical transformations, thereby forming energy. Each cell, in this case, is a miniature power station. Interestingly, the number of mitochondria in each cell depends on the energy requirements. With regular exercise, it increases, to provide greater production of the necessary energy. Conversely, a sedentary lifestyle leads to a decrease in energy production and, accordingly, a decrease in the number of mitochondria. Different nutrients are needed to convert to energy, each of which causes various stages of the process energy. Therefore, consumption of food should be not only nourishing but also contain all kinds of nutrients needed to produce energy: carbohydrates, proteins, and fats.

It is very important to restore the content in the ration products, take energy, or hinder its education. All similar products stimulate adrenaline hormone emissions.

For the normal functioning of the body, it is important to maintain a constant level of glucose in the blood. For this purpose, it is desirable to give preference to food with a low glycemic index. By adding protein and fiber to every meal or snack, you are thereby contributing to the accumulation of enough energy.

Carbohydrates and Glucose

Energy, which we extract from food, comes mostly from carbohydrates rather than proteins or fats. Carbohydrates are more easily converted to glucose and are therefore the most convenient source of energy for the body.

Glucose can be spent on energy needs immediately, or delayed as a reserve in the liver and muscles. It is stored in the form of glycogen, which, if necessary, is easily converted into it again. With the "fight or run" syndrome (see), glycogen is released into the bloodstream to provide the body with additional energy. Glycogen is stored in soluble form.

Proteins Must Be Balanced with Carbohydrates

Although carbohydrates and proteins are essential for everyone, their ratios can fluctuate depending on individual needs and habits. The optimum ratio is adjusted individually by trial and error, but you can be guided by data.

Be careful with proteins. Always add high-quality complex carbohydrates, such as dense vegetables or cereal grains, to them. The predominance of protein foods leads to acidification of the internal environment of the body, while it should be slightly alkaline. The internal system of self-regulation allows the body to return to an alkalized state through the release of calcium from bones. Ultimately, this can disrupt the bone structure, lead to osteoporosis, in which fractures often occur.

Useful Advice

Health drinks and snacks, containing glucose, provide quick energy, but this effect is fleeting. Moreover, it is accompanied by a depletion of the body's energy reserves. During sports, you spend a lot of energy. Therefore, you can "refuel" soybean curds with fresh berries in front of them.

What Is Necessary for You (Protein/Carbohydrate Ratio)

- PASSIVE
  A man in his old age, bedridden, 1: 2 recovering

- NOT VERY ACTIVE
  Official, owner of a small 1: 1.5 store, housewife

- ACTIVE
  Man, regularly engaged in 1: 1.25 in sports, working mother, student

- VERY ACTIVE
  Athlete or bodybuilder, 1: 1 ballet dancer

Try a little bit to increase protein intake, while reducing the amount of carbohydrates, or vice versa, until you determine the optimum power level for yourself.

Energy Needs Throughout Life

The need for additional energy arises in us at various stages of life. In childhood, for example, energy is necessary for growth and learning in adolescence—to ensure hormonal and physical changes during puberty. During pregnancy, the need for energy increases as the mother and the fetus, and during stress, excess energy expended throughout life. In addition, a person leading an active lifestyle needs more energy than ordinary people.

Energy Plunders

It is very important to limit the content in the diet of foods that take energy or prevent its formation. Such products include alcohol, tea, coffee, and fizzy drinks, as well as cakes, biscuits, and sweets. All such products stimulate the release of the adrenaline hormone, which is formed in the adrenal glands. The fastest way adrenaline is formed by the so-called syndrome of "beysya or flight" when we that—is threatened. The adrenaline rush mobilizes the body to action. The heart begins to beat quickened, the lungs absorb more air, the liver releases glucose into the bloodstream longer, and the blood flows back, where it is needed—for example, to the feet. Constantly increased adrenaline formation, in particular, with appropriate nutrition, can lead to an enduring feeling of fatigue.

Stress is also considered one of the energy plunders, since stress releases the stored glucose from the liver and muscles, which leads to a short-term burst of energy, followed by a state of prolonged fatigue.

Energy and Emotions

In the "fight or run" syndrome, glycogen (stored carbohydrates) enters the liver from the bloodstream, which leads to an increase in the level of sugar in it. In view of this, prolonged stressful conditions can seriously affect blood sugar levels. Caffeine and nicotine have a similar effect; the latter contribute to the secretion of two hormones— cortisone and adrenaline, which interfere with the digestion process and cause the liver to throw out stored glycogen.

45

Food Rich in Energy

The richest in terms of energy are the products containing vitamins B complex: In 1, In 2, In 3, B 5, B 6, B 12, B 9 (folic acid), and biotin. All of them are abundant in grains of millet, buckwheat, rye, quinoa (a South—American herb, is very popular in the West), corn, and barley. In sprouting grains, the energy value increases many times—the nutritional value of the seedlings is increased by the enzymes that promote growth. Many types of vitamin B are also found in fresh herbs.

Vitamin C, which is present in fruits (for example, oranges) and vegetables (potatoes, peppers), is also important for the body's energy; magnesium, which is abundant in greens, nuts, and seeds; zinc (egg yolk, fish, sunflower seeds); iron (grains, pumpkin seeds, lentils); copper (shell of Brazil nut, oats, salmon, mushrooms), as well as coenzyme Q10, which is present in beef, sardines, spinach and peanuts.

Maintaining Normal Blood Sugar

How often did you have to wake up in the morning in a bad mood, feeling lethargy, overwhelming, and experiencing the urgent need to sleep for another hour—another? And life seems no joy. Or, perhaps, tormented before noon, you wonder, and will make it there before lunch. Even worse, when fatigue overcomes you after dinner at the end of the day, and you have no idea how to get home. And there, after all, you still have to cook dinner. And then—to eat. And do not you ask yourself: "Lord, where has my strength disappeared?"

Persistent fatigue and lack of energy can be caused by various reasons, but most often they are the result of poor diets and/or irregular nutrition, as well as abuse of stimulants that help to "hold out".

Depression, irritability, and mood swings, in addition to premenstrual syndrome, outbreaks of anger, excitement, and nervousness can be the result of an imbalance in the process of energy formation, malnutrition, and frequent sitting on fancy diets.

Get an idea, how and from which energy is produced in our body, we can in a short time to increase their power, which will not only continue to operate and a good mood throughout the day, but will also provide a healthy deep sleep at night.

Glucose is not the normal sugar molecule, obtained when the enzymatic digestion of proteins, fats, and carbohydrates. The structure is a complex sugar in contrast to conventional sugar, which is added to the granola, effervescent beverages, cakes, and biscuits.

Energy Food

All foods can be divided into three classes, depending on the energy supplied by the body. The most effective products are class 1. Class 2 products also give us a lot of energy but are inferior in this respect to Class 1 products. Finally, products of class 3 serve as sources of "cheap" energy—you experience a quick energy surge, but it does not last long. If you feel the need for additional energy resources, then arrange themselves during the day small pause to stay one's stomach with the help of products containing carbohydrates and proteins 1 and 2 classes.

Class 1 Products

- **Complex Carbohydrates**
  Grains of oats, barley, brown rice, millet, whole grain bread, rye bread, cornbread

- **Vegetables**
  Dense vegetables, such as broccoli, cauliflower, Brussels

sprouts; mushrooms, turnips, carrots (especially—damp), asparagus, artichokes, spinach

- **Fruits**
  Avocado, apples, pears, pineapple, berries—strawberries, raspberries, black currants, cherries

- **Protein**
  Salmon, tuna, herring, mackerel, seaweed, eggs, tofu, walnuts, Brazil nuts, sunflower seeds, pumpkins, sesame seeds, flax. Seedlings of seeds and grains, green beans and lima beans, mutton chickpeas, lentils, and soybeans.

Class 2 Products

- **Complex Carbohydrates**
  Buckwheat, red macrobiotic rice, Canadian rice, oatmeal cakes

- **Vegetables**
  Potatoes, sweet potatoes, corn, pumpkin, beets, peppers, Canadian rice, yams, watercress—lettuce, leaf lettuce

- **Fruits**
  Peaches, Apricots, Mango, Papaya, Banana

- **Protein**
  Common beans, dried peas, almonds, chicken, wild bird,

turkey, venison, peanut butter, yogurt, cottage cheese, fish

Grade 3 Products

- **Carbohydrates**
  Pasta, bread, rice, rice noodles, egg noodles

- **Vegetables**
  Tomatoes, green peas, zucchini, cucumbers

- **Fruits**
  Prunes, any dried fruits, grapes, figs

- **Proteins**
  Dairy products, such as cheese and milk, red meat, duck, veal

Carbohydrates are considered the best source of "fuel" for the body, as they are converted to glucose with the greatest ease. However, the food which is too rich in carbohydrates can upset the delicate balance of blood sugar levels, causing it to significant fluctuations. Better balance all carbohydrates, add food, containing fiber, protein, and a small amount of fat.

After the digestion of food and the entry of nutrients into the bloodstream, the pancreas under the action of hormones begins to secrete insulin, through which glucose is transported through cell membranes. If the level of sugar (glucose) in the blood exceeds the needs of the body, the excess goes to the liver, where it is stored in reserve.

However, if blood sugar rises too quickly, the pancreas begins to secrete excess insulin. This explains the sudden changes in the state of health, which are experienced by many people when, how sweet a treat. Chocolate bar invigorates well, providing quick energy, but pretty soon people, it ate, begins to feel more sluggish than before the meal. This impact of the pancreas is called "reactive hypoglycemia". For a long period, if you do not change the diet, it can lead to the development of diabetes.

Useful Advice

Stimulating drinks, like tea or coffee, have a stressful effect on the body, contributing only to a short-term flow of energy. It is better to replace them with either green tea, which contains little caffeine and has antioxidant properties, or diluted orange juice.

The formation and secretion of insulin by the pancreas is stimulated by the combined action of vitamin B 3 (niacin) and chromium. People who suffer from reactive hypoglycemia, as well as malnourished, often exhibit a lack of chromium in the body.

Insidious Sugar

Sugar is the most malicious violator of the energy production process in the body. And—very insidious. After all, it is found not only in obvious sweets—sweets, cakes, and carbonated drinks—but it is present in hidden form in many finished products, sauces, breakfast cereals, bread, and pizza. Sugar is truly omnipresent.

To determine the daily amount of sugar consumed, pay attention to the label. All ingredients are listed in descending order of content. On a chocolate bar, for example, you will see immediately, that sugar tops the list, while cocoa is significantly lower. There is even a natural question—what kind of tile are they offering us, chocolate, or sugar? And looking closely at the labels of almost all prepared foods, you will see that sugar is almost always present. It is logical to ask, why add sugar in certain food? If you yourself, while preparing this dish at home, do not put sugar, then why do manufacturers? The answer is simple: add sugar because of its relatively low cost, as well as its ability to give this product a familiar (or, allegedly, even better) taste. However, we nutritionists insist that adding sugar to foods is completely useless.

Sugar in the Morning, Sugar in the Evening

Often, we cannot imagine how much we consume sugar, because it can be there, where no one that does not expect.

Here, let's say, a typical daily diet for a Westerner. Breakfast: granola, toast, and coffee. Of the three components of the sugar contained, at least two, or even all three: dry breakfast bread, and he is always there, but in the coffee, you add it to taste yourself. The same is true for the second breakfast, consisting of a pair of biscuits and cans of juice or soda. If lunch includes a sandwich, bread, and some—a drink at the bank, then, in all likelihood, the sugar will be present everywhere. Mid-morning snack, consisting of biscuits and chocolates with tea, also bring your sugar mite. And even for dinner, the menu of which includes pasta with bottled sauce or a "ready-to-eat" dish, a fair amount of sugar is provided for sure.

You will be surprised if you know how much hidden sugar in foods that we traditionally refer to the "healthy": in yogurt, many fruit juices, canned beans, and other vegetables. Even sugar, contained in natural products, such as honey or molasses (molasses), could seriously undermine the normal balance of blood sugar. All such products contribute to raising its level, disrupt the normal secretion of insulin, and expose the body to stress.

To protect yourself from sugar, perform the following experiment: for two weeks, avoid sugar at anything. Do not add it to tea and coffee, refuse chocolate, honey, and other sweets, announce a boycott for desserts. After two weeks, try to swallow a teaspoon of sugar—the taste will seem so sweet to you, so unbearably sweet.

Alcohol, in any form, acts like simple sugars, and, being absorbed directly from the stomach, enters the bloodstream. That's why booze on an empty stomach has an intoxicating effect so quickly: alcohol enters the brain, breaks it, and the ability to soberly assess the situation (in particular, if you're driving), causing ataxia. Before you take a nip, you should certainly have something to eat—this will slow the flow of alcohol into the bloodstream. But to drive tipsy—a flagrant violation of matter, they ate it or not.

Fruits, especially eaten on an empty stomach, as a rule, are digested very quickly. But they can affect blood sugar levels in the same way as regular sugar, although to a lesser extent. That's why people that exhibit mood swings, vitality, and well-being, it is not necessary to follow a diet, according to which fruit should be eaten only until noon. Although fruits are effective antioxidants and a good source of fiber, consume them should, observing moderation. If you have trouble maintaining normal levels of sugar, then, perhaps, the fruit is best avoided altogether.

The most effective way to maintain normal sugar levels in the blood is to eliminate sugar and to make sure that every meal includes proteins. Proteins promote hormone secretion, which slows down the release of carbohydrates. An ideal source of protein is nuts, beans, and beans, tofu, eggs, fish, and poultry. For example, after you eat a plate of pasta with ketchup, your blood sugar will jump up sharply, but will soon drop again. If you add to this dish of tofu or chicken, the digestive process is slowed down, and the blood sugar level will not change significantly. Proteins should be combined with fiber, which also slows the formation of sugars during digestion and helps control blood sugar.

Some foods break down to carbohydrate levels quickly, while others are much slower. It is preferable to use the latter for nutrition. Each product has a so-called "glycemic index", the higher which, the faster the carbohydrates contained in this product will raise blood sugar. However, you must remember that in the freshly squeezed juice of raw vegetables, example: carrots, glycemic index rises sharply due to the lack of fiber in juice, slowing down the process of digestion. The table lists the products, differing in glycemic index.

Glycemic Index

All products have a different glycemic index. The most useful are those whose glycemic levels range from low to medium; carbohydrates at the same time come slowly, and the blood sugar level does not undergo significant fluctuations. But try to avoid foods with a high glycemic index. They not only contribute to a sharp rise in blood sugar levels but rather quickly deplete the stored energy by the body, causing you to feel tired more pronounced than before.

High Glycemic Index
- honey
- drinks in cans
- chocolate and other sweets
- white rice and rice cakes
- French loaves
- cornflakes
- baked potato
- raisins
- apricots

- dried fruits
- roots, past the cooking process

Medium Glycemic Index

- popcorn
- corn chips
- brown rice
- pasta
- bagels

Low Glycemic Index

- Rye bread
- yogurt (sugar-free)
- cereal grains (millet, buckwheat, brown rice, quinoa)
- legumes (beans and beans, lentils, lamb chickpeas)
- apples
- pears
- any raw root vegetables

Healthy Sleep—Victory with Insomnia

Many of us tend to complain of insomnia from time to time, but some people suffer from it constantly, and as a result, they feel overwhelmed, irritable, and become less efficient. To restore strength, the body needs a normal sleep. At night, under the influence of human growth hormone, proteins build new cells, find and repair damage. This hormone is secreted only during sleep, so for normal functioning, the body needs night or day rest.

Stress and any stimulants (alcohol, tea, coffee, various colas, chocolate, and stimulating drugs), both, however, and dense foods before bedtime, indigestion, and unstable blood sugar levels disrupt normal sleep. In view of this, if you notice that you begin to sleep badly, note when and how you dine.

Energy-Boosting Snacks

These healthy snacks are ideal for maintaining blood sugar throughout the day.

- Almonds, dates, and apples
- Dried fruits (their consumption should be limited to 1-2 times a week) and a handful of different nuts
- Natural nonfat yogurt (sugar-free) with chopped pumpkin seeds and wheat seedlings
- Oatcakes with wheat seedlings and dried apricots
- Crispbread or Oatmeal Cheese Cakes
- Cream—sauce with avocado and rice bread
- Raw vegetables with yogurt or cream—with sour cream sauce
- Breakfast cereal (granola) without sugar, with nuts and dried fruits
- Hummus with crispbread or oatmeal cakes
- Fruits with Sesame Seeds

Answer these questions, and you will learn how stable is the sugar level in your blood.

If the level of blood sugar rises quickly, this will entail its subsequent sharp fall, as well as the release of insulin, causing you to feel tired and start to feel the need for some—a stimulator. The sharp rises and drops in blood sugar have a negative effect on our well-being and energy. The key to excellent health is the ability to restore normal blood sugar levels.

1. Do you think that 7 hours of night sleep is not enough for your body?

2. Do you feel lethargic and heavy in the morning?
3. Do you feel the need to start the day with something—something exciting (tea, coffee, cigarette)?
4. Do you regularly drink tea and coffee throughout the day?
5. Do you tend to drink carbonated drinks throughout the day?
6. Do you have frequent urination?
7. Do your palms sweat?
8. Do you smoke?
9. Do you look forward, the evening drink that—something strong?
10. Does it happen that when you feel thirsty, it is not quenched even after drinking water?
11. Do you feel sleepy during the day?
12. Do you want to during the day to eat sweet, taste of bread or any other food, rich in carbohydrates?
13. Do you happen to abandon the charge of the–of the feeling of fatigue?
14. Do you tend to from time to time to notice that you cannot concentrate?
15. Do you feel dizzy or irritation, if you cannot eat often?

If you answered "yes" to three questions and more, it is quite possible that your body has difficulty in maintaining a stable blood sugar level. Try to follow our advice and check whether there is an improvement.

If you answered "yes" more than five questions, the difficulty in maintaining a stable level of blood sugar, you would almost certainly experience. Follow our recommendations. If improvement does not follow, contact your doctor and/or nutritionist for further examination.

Products containing saturated fatty acids, for example, dairy products, meat, and hard cheese are digested in a relatively long time, so it is desirable to avoid their use for dinner. Instead, it is preferable to use fried fish and vegetables, rice, and salads, since they carry a much lower burden on the digestive system. After dinner, instead of caffeinated tea or coffee, it is good to drink herbal tea with mint (stimulates digestion) and chamomile (relaxes).

Useful Advice

Dinner, consisting of fish with herbs, will give you deep sleep because it contains a lot of calcium and magnesium, which are necessary to ensure stable brain activity, as well as to relax the muscles of the body.

Products containing tyramine, an amino acid, which is present in vegetables of the nightshade family (tomatoes, eggplant, zucchini, potatoes), as well as in spinach, stimulate the secretion of adrenaline, which can lead to a disturbance in normal sleep. Tyramine is also found in alcohol, bacon, ham, and sausage, so it is advisable to limit the consumption of these products for dinner.

Calcium and magnesium are mineral substances necessary for normal sleep. The lack of any of them can lead to insomnia. If you have disturbed sleep, eat more foods containing these elements, and your sleep must be improved. We recommend adding broccoli, cauliflower, Brussels sprouts, mackerel, peas, chicken, salmon, greens, and cabbage to the menu of your dinner.

Another amino acid, tryptophan, is produced in the brain to regulate sleep. Many tryptophans contain bananas, turkey, tuna, figs, dates, peanut butter, and whole-wheat crackers. Add any of these products to your dinner or try them at night, and you have a good night 's sleep.

PMS—Monthly Torture

Not every woman suffers from premenstrual syndrome (PMS), but those, the share of which falls this meal, do not know where to find refuge from the monsters, which is tear their flesh with alarming frequency. For some women, the inconvenience associated with PMS is purely physical in nature. They experience pain in the lower part of the pelvis, the mammary glands swell and become rough, swelling is observed. Sometimes women experience a serious decline in well-being.

But for other women, PMS marks the onset of a real emotional crisis, comparable, for example, with imprisonment. Moreover, alarming symptoms can appear both in the middle of the cycle, and several days before the onset of menstruation. Such women are characterized not only by irritability, causeless outbursts of anger, and sudden mood swings but sometimes, they can even be visited by thoughts of suicide. Moreover, the sufferers are completely unable to keep themselves in control and often become closed and uncommunicative. These women sometimes explain their own behavior as follows: "as if a stranger had settled in my head", and often they themselves are amazed at their actions. As a rule, attentive husbands and friends succeed in time to see these symptoms and understand what they are called.

Hormonal Balance

One of the main causes of PMS is an imbalance in the hormones of estrogen and progesterone. Although its origin can be "natural" character, without the interference of external factors, the causes of PMS are few.

Every day we come across various products and products (for example, plastic containers and wrappers) that have an estrogen-like effect and are able to change the normal level of estrogen in the body. Usually, the amount of estrogen decreases in the middle of the cycle, while the level of progesterone, on the contrary, increases (progesterone is a hormone that helps maintain pregnancy), and therefore excess estrogen can upset this delicate balance.

Another reason, contributing to the development of PMS, is a disruption of the normal level of sugar in the blood, which may, in turn, be caused by immoderate eating sugar, simple carbohydrates, and foods, past technological processing. In addition, high levels of sugar consumption deplete the body of magnesium, a mineral substance, needed for muscle relaxation. That is why there is menstrual pain, and cramps can be overcome, adding to the diet food, rich in magnesium: grain cereals, leafy greens, dairy products, fish, and seafood.

Complex B vitamins are also needed for relaxation, reducing chest pain, and swelling, supporting the adrenal glands, and controlling stress. Whole grains of cereals are good sources of B vitamins: millet, rye, buckwheat, and brown rice.

PMS and Craving for Food

Before the onset of menstruation, many women have a craving for various foods. Most often, women are attracted by stimulants such as tea, coffee, and alcohol, which disrupt normal blood sugar levels, alter the secretion of the stress hormone and, as a result, lead to mood swings. You can deal with such cravings by frequent meals of small amounts of food throughout the day.

Useful Advice

If at night you can't fall asleep for a long time, do not despair—get up and eat some dates with a slice of banana, or try low-fat yogurt with a teaspoon of peanut butter. Better yet, mix all of the listed ingredients a little bit into a "midnight cocktail."

Before menstruation, many women are drawn to feast on chocolate. The reason is that chocolate contains a lot of magnesium, and it provides a quick influx of energy due to an imbalance in blood sugar. However, the body is more useful to give preference to other products containing magnesium, for example, apricots, figs, and peaches, which will satisfy the most exacting taste without any adverse effects. To correct blood sugar levels, it is good to add a protein source to these products, for example, almonds (also contains magnesium) and other nuts or seeds.

Is Your Child a Fidgety One or a Quiet One?

The reasons for excessive childhood activity are several. Some are hereditary or associated with the environment in which the child grows but still dominated by the dependence of the nervous system from the diet.

Classic symptoms include an excessive activity of an inability to focus on any game or other activity for more than a few minutes; violent bursts of energy, followed by exhaustion; "butting", aggressiveness towards other children (and adults); excessive moodiness and irritability.

Products That Improve Memory and Concentration

No matter, whether you are preparing for the exam, spend 10 hours of the office, arrange the reception, sit behind the wheel of a car, or perform any other work, requiring concentration and intense mental activity, these processes are directly dependent on your food consumption throughout the day.

For the normal functioning of brain cells, choline, one of the B vitamins, is needed. Once in the brain, it is converted to acetylcholine, a neurotransmitter that transfers information between brain cells. A low level of acetylcholine leads to impaired memory—from "the language turns, but I can't remember" to its complete loss. Choline is also required to form and maintain the integrity of the myelin sheath, which protects nerve cells and promotes the rapid and accurate transmission of information.

There are a number of products rich in choline including veal liver, cauliflower, caviar, eggs, lentils, and soy products.

For the formation of another neurotransmitter, dopamine, essential vitamin B 3, and iron are essential. Dopamine is involved in the formation and maintenance of memory. Good sources of vitamin B 3 are brewer's yeast, turkey meat, halibut, pumpkin seeds, and peanuts. For products, rich in iron, include veal liver, apricots (especially apricots), raisins, pumpkin seeds, and walnuts.

To maintain memory, all B complex vitamins are needed (B 1, B 2, B 3, B 5, B 6, B 12, biotin and B 9, folic acid). With a deficiency of these vitamins, memory loss, impaired concentration, impaired perception, and general forgetfulness are noted. Vitamin B complex is also needed for the production of cellular energy, and especially—in the brain cells.

The most useful foods include brewer's yeast, chicken, leafy cabbage, cabbage, oatmeal, soybeans, fish, avocados, and potatoes.

A child may be uncomfortable with his awkwardness, injustice at food, inattention in school. Moreover, all attempts to achieve his perseverance and attention, as a rule, end in failure.

To overcome excessive childhood activity, you can use the method of proper nutrition. Children respond quickly to changes in diet, and you'll quickly realize what products have a negative impact on the child's behavior. To do this, it is enough for several weeks to remove one or another food product from the child's diet, and then return it again.

In order to determine the value of certain products, in the first step, you need to keep a food diary. To control changes in the behavior of the child, it is necessary to remove from his diet all sweetened foods, drinks with fruit additives, effervescent and fruit drinks, as well as all products that are processed and ready to eat. Any food containing dyes, additives, and a lot of sugar is able to have a negative impact on the brain and behavior of the child.

In addition, shown, that is naturally found in some food's salicylates (components, acting like aspirin), are perhaps the main culprits of disorders of the brain centers, responsible for the child's behavior. Often, we are convinced that it is enough to remove from the diet of a child citrus fruits and orange juice, to the child's behavior has changed dramatically for the better.

Polyunsaturated fatty acids, which are necessary for the transmission of nerve impulses, also play an important role in the management of childhood injustice. Their lack of or even imbalance can disrupt the transfer of information from one nerve ending to another. A diet high in sugar may interfere with the proper disposal of polyunsaturated fatty acids, which would entail malfunctions and errors in the transmission of nerve impulses. At excessively active children often exhibit a lack of polyunsaturated omega -3 fatty acids, as a consequence, it is recommended to add such products in the diet of children, containing them. These include oily fish (tuna, sardines, salmon, mackerel), as well as pumpkin and sunflower oils (they should be used for salads and dressing, but not for cooking hot food).

The diet of restless children is often lacking leafy vegetable culture, containing magnesium. Their absence leads to a violation of the delicate balance of calcium and magnesium, necessary for the optimal functioning of the brain and nervous system. To normalize the level of magnesium in the body, it is advisable to add broccoli, green peas, cauliflower, spinach, figs, as well as cereal grains, including oats and brown rice, to children's diet.

There are other possible causes of overly active behavior of children. If the above tips to change the power of the child, had no significant effect on the change in his behavior, you should suspect a harmful influence of the environment, or the consequences of—or toxic effects. It is advisable to consult with appropriate specialists. In particular, the toxicologist can conduct accurate tests. Other causes include physical injury, such as a fall, which could result in some kind of disturbance that is not visible from the outside. Our advice—do not neglect the advice of professionals.

Dealing with Stress

"Stress"—a word, hackneyed to the limit, but do you know exactly what does it mean? In order to function normally, our body is constantly striving to maintain all physiological processes in dynamic equilibrium. Stress—is any impact, which is the equilibrium is disturbed. The body has to defend itself with great difficulty from the physical and emotional stress to which it is constantly exposed.

Stress is an unavoidable evil, manifested in many forms. It is hard to imagine life without stress; each at one time or another, every one of us is subjected to stress. There are two types of stress—external and internal. External (exogenous) stress factors, the most familiar to us, affect the body from the outside. Internal (endogenous) factors act from the depths of our bodies. Descriptions of both types of stress are given in the plate on the right.

To understand, what exactly is the detrimental effects of stress on the body, you must look into the past. The survival of the primitive man depended primarily on his luck on the hunt and on the ability to avoid the claws and fangs of predators. With the threat of attack, our body instantly throws in the bloodstream stress hormones, which contribute to the energy supply to the organs, on which our protection and rescue depend. This is the so-called "fight or run" reaction. Although in our time, we are rarely attacked by predatory animals; nevertheless, the physiological reaction to the danger threatening the body has remained from the time of Adam. When stress hormones are released, the brain immediately enters a state of alert, and the organs of all five senses begin to function at an exacerbated level.

When the body responds to stressful effects, significant changes occur in it, each of which is a continuation of the "fight or run" syndrome. They can be divided into seven main types.

1. The pulse quickens, and the heart pumps more blood to enhance the transport of nutrients needed to produce additional energy.

2. Breathing quickens to enrich the blood with oxygen and increases the excretion of carbon dioxide.

3. The blood vessels that supply blood to the brain and muscles expand, which contributes to the increased flow of oxygen, glucose, and nutrients to them.

4. Increased supply to the functioning of the spleen, increased influx of lymphocytes. It increases blood clotting, in the case of injury.

5. To increase energy, the liver and skeletal muscles release an additional amount of glucose into the blood.

6. Pupils dilate, and more light enters the eye, which helps to improve vision.

7. The digestion process slows down, the production of digestive enzymes stops, as a result of which more energy is released for the muscles and the brain.

Thus, the "fight or flight" complex of reactions prepares the body for targeted active actions for a short time. A too-long stay of an organism in a state of combat readiness has a harmful effect on health and the psyche. For comparison, try, sitting in the car, put the lever shift to "neutral" by simultaneously pressing the accelerator pedal and the brake!

In such cases, the body tries to return to the usual state of harmonic balance, for which it changes its settings, adapting to stress. For example, the body can arbitrarily increase blood pressure or dramatically reduce the concentration of glucose in the blood.

Standing stress effect leads to the fact that we live "on the nerves"— and we are wasting precious energy reserves.

But back to our ancestors. After prolonged stress, they gave the body a break, allowing it to restore balance. The symptoms of the "fight or run" complex faded away, normal levels of hormones, blood sugar were restored, digestion normalized. The modern pace of life often leaves us no such luxury, as the recovery time.

There are so many stresses in our lives—and often they are so lasting— that the body is almost in a state of "fight or run" without respite. And, as a result, we constantly live "on the nerves", wasting precious, precious reserves of glucose and energy. Once the body to recover, which may, ultimately, lead to physiological changes. The most common physiological effects of stress are listed below. In addition to this, some types of food can have an additional stressful effect on an already overloaded body, contributing to the depletion of energy resources.

Symptoms of stress—physiological effects of stress:

- Suppression of the immune system, leading to an increase in colds and infectious diseases
- Craving for a certain type of food
- Weight loss

- Constant fatigue
- Loss of appetite
- Dramatic mood swings
- Depressed state
- Excitement
- Skin rash

How to Assess Emotional Stress

Curiously, that the emotional distress felt by all—differently. The fact which is an absolute stress for you, someone else may have paid no attention to it. The stress in any situation can be reduced if you force yourself to evaluate it from a different point of view. Take, for example, public speaking, which many are scared of. For the first time, they may well cause a stressful reaction: sweating of the palms, an adrenaline rush. But already at the second or third public appearance, these reactions, as a rule, are dulled, and the speaker copes with his task with much greater peace of mind. Accordingly, stress is also reduced. But the situation has remained the same—only its perception has changed. If you accustom yourself to treat stress as inevitable, then coping with it becomes easier.

Food as a Stress Factor

Food, not very useful for the body, or cause allergies, can cause stress. In addition, digestive disorders, caused by malnutrition, bacterial, or parasitic infection, can lead to increased intestinal wall permeability, whereby the bloodstream particles will fall junk food. As a result, an immune response will develop, which, with frequent repetitions, will increase the load on the adrenal glands. That is, a situation arises "tricks -22", when the adrenal glands in response to stress will allocate more cortisone, which, in turn, seeks to redress the balance. One of the negative aspects of excess cortisone is digestion. This cycle repeats over and over, and ultimately inevitably affects health.

An optimistic attitude towards life also helps to reduce the harmful effects of stress. For example, you're stuck in traffic, so what? It's not your fault, so you can relax, listen to music, or chat with your companion. Do everything, it depends on you, call on his cell phone to the service and explain, why linger. If you can't change the situation, then take it for granted.

Stress, Food, and Nutrients

So, what do we do? If we can't influence the majority of external stressors in any way, then we are quite capable of helping our bodies cope with their manifestations.

Some nutrients, for example, not only help in coping with stress but also support the functions of the bodies involved in the stress response. So, say, the "magnificent five"—vitamins A, C, E, as well as trace elements zinc and selenium—successfully neutralize free radicals that are formed in the body under the influence of stress. Among food products containing these vital antioxidants include plums, tomatoes, kiwi fruit, dark-green vegetables, seafood, sesame seeds, and pumpkin.

Stress and the Immune System

It is well known that people, under stress, the most prone to disease. This is due to the fact that stress weakens the immune system. When stressful effects increase, we often suffer from colds and infectious diseases, and in the most severe cases, our immune system does not cope with a precancerous state, as it would during a period of rest and carelessness. The state of combat readiness lowers the body's resistance to infections since it treats them as a lesser evil compared to the danger in this case. As a result, the activity of killer cells is inhibited, the T-system of immunity is disrupted, and infectious agents feel at ease. Therefore, it is obvious that during stress it is necessary to stimulate the immune system.

Hormones of the Immune System

In times of stress, a balance of two hormones is vital to maintaining the immune system. This is Dehydroepiandosterone (DHEA) and cortisone. Scientists have shown that many people, suffering from chronic diseases, DHEA levels are low, and vice versa—significantly elevated cortisol levels (the amount of these hormones can be easily measured with a simple saliva test). Reasons, which falls DHEA content, several. Under the influence of stress, the adrenal glands cease to secrete DHEA and switch to cortisone. The resulting imbalance has on the body as a negative impact, as well as suppression of the immune system. DHEA levels decline with age, and in 70-80 years in our body it is made five times less than in adolescence and early adulthood. A decrease in the level of this hormone depends on body fat (especially around the waist), constant hunger, insomnia, lack of sex drive, and a tendency to allergies and infectious diseases.

If any of these items tend to you, ask your adviser—a nutritionist or physician to make an analysis on the content you take—DHEA and cortisone.

Useful Advice

When under stress, try to avoid coffee and tea, replacing them with diluted fruit or vegetable juices. They will supply your body with vitamin C and magnesium necessary for health, the amount of which decreases under stress.

If it turns out that their level is low, then restoring the normal DHEA content will allow you not only to lower cholesterol but also to strengthen the skeleton and improve the ratio of muscle tissue to fat. But the second hormone, cortisone, is potentially dangerous. An increase in its content can lead to a disorder of the thyroid gland and joints, leading to a decrease in energy. Moreover, with a high level of cortisone, a violation of the structure of muscle and bone tissue occurs, which can lead to osteoporosis.

Some food products have stress influence on the organism. Stress can be caused by the lack of any nutrient as that negatively impacts on dependence on them enzymatic processes.

How to increase DHEA levels and reduce the content of cortisone so that the equilibrium of DHEA and cortisol can be restored?

Supporting the adrenal glands with the recommended anti-stress products as well as by relaxing through meditation or yoga exercises. In the most severe cases, caused by prolonged stress, the adrenal glands reduce the secretion of both DHEA and cortisol. This condition is called adrenal insufficiency or a crisis.

In such cases, it is desirable to compensate for the lack of both hormones by means of dosed supplements of licorice rhizome and Siberian ginseng. However, this can only be done under the supervision of a professional nutritionist.

In the US supplements, containing in its composition DHEA, you can buy not only in pharmacies but also in some stores selling healthy food. However, in some countries, DHEA or its predecessor pregnenolone, which has a similar effect, can be prescribed—only a doctor can do so.

Fighting Stress with Nutrition

So how do you all—still cope with stress? Although it is not in our power to counteract some external stressors, however, we can radically change how the diet of their food, and their own way of life.

Some foods have a stressful effect on the body. Stress is also a lack of any—any nutrient, because of their lack of a negative impact on their dependent enzymatic processes. To support adrenal function, the body needs vitamin B 5, vitamin C, and magnesium. To combat the effects of daily stress, you need every day to include in your diet enough food containing these vitamins and minerals. For the normal functioning of the adrenal vitamin C must be a lot, and it is the only vitamin, which is not stored in our body as a reserve—we have to get it from food daily. Most vitamin C is found in all red and blackberries, kiwi fruits, and citrus fruits, as well as in potatoes and peppers. All this can be purchased at any supermarket.

During a period of increased stress, the need for these vitamins increases many times. One of the most common signs of vitamin C deficiency is stomatitis or ulceration of the mucous membranes of the oral cavity. By normalizing vitamin C intake, you can get rid of unpleasant sores in just 24 hours.

Stress Fighters

On a busy day, only a few can afford to do a little breathing room, so, slowly, to taste healthy foods. For busy people, we recommend cooking in the morning and taking with you the service nutritious mini-snacks, which during the day can be intercepted literally "on the run".

Smoked salmon paste on whole-grain crackers, Rye toast with almond oil, Spinach salad with sunflower seeds, etc.

Magnesium is necessary for the normal functioning of the adrenal glands, so foods high in magnesium should be present daily in your diet. These are cereal grains, greens, soybeans, wheat germ, almonds, cod, and mackerel. In whole grains of cereals, in leafy greens, as well as in meat and dairy products, there is a lot of vitamin B 5.

Of course, the availability of products, the opposing stress, implies the existence of such products, which are, on the contrary, contribute to it. Thus, abuse of sugar and refined carbohydrates leads to the depletion of many essential trace elements, in particular, magnesium, and also affects the pancreas, forcing her to increased insulin secretion (see. Maintaining normal blood sugar levels,). For some time out—for the functioning of the pancreas, increased load is disrupted, which in some cases leads to an early manifestation of adult diabetes.

Reducing or completely eliminating sugar from the diet has an extremely beneficial effect on the liver increases its function in the neutralization of toxic substances. The liver is the main organ—a cleaner in the body. Its role is to continuously filter the blood and remove all potentially toxic substances, as well as slag, formed as a result of normal digestion. Therefore, any reduction in the stress load on the liver affects its basic function in the most beneficial way. Keep in mind that such stimulants, such as tea, coffee, and alcoholic drinks deplete certain trace elements and stimulate the production of adrenaline; therefore, reducing the consumption of these drinks will also allow you to deal with stress more effectively.

Obviously, it should be limited or even completely eliminate from your diet refined and stored for a long time "ready to eat" products, which contain lots of artificial preservatives, salt, sugar, and have very low nutritional value.

Plan to deal with stress on a weekend. In order to feel the surge of energy, and in order, to get a little to relieve his impossibly zastressovanny body, select a couple of days when you cannot afford to bother too much. Store plenty of fresh fruits, vegetables, and mineral water. Punish yourself for the weekend to eat only raw food: from it, you will gather an abundance of nutrients needed to deal with stress.

Every morning, start with 3 cups of warm boiled water. You can add a slice of lemon or 2-3 slices of fresh raw ginger to enhance its aroma, however, drink water strictly on an empty stomach. This tonic drink has a beneficial effect on your liver and stimulates the outflow of bile. This is especially useful if the day before you allowed yourself to indulgence in food or abused alcohol.

You can squeeze juice from almost all vegetables and fruits. Try to drink fresh juice from herbs 3-4 times daily. For the preparation of vegetable juices are best suited:

- cress-salad
- parsley
- spinach
- zucchini
- green pepper
- leaf lettuce

Since fruits are very rich in fructose, it is advisable to dilute fruit juices with water in half before use.

Try to relax better, go for a walk, sleep enough. Probably, on Sunday, you will feel a mild headache, or you will have muscle ache, but it is— a good sign, testifying to the fact that your body is cleaned. Remember that even at the beginning of next week, you will feel such freshness as if you were on vacation! And do not forget to drink more water for the whole weekend. You can also go for an acupressure or aromatherapy session—combine business with pleasure in the process of body cleansing.

Soya milkshake with fresh berries, Potato salad with herring rollups, Strawberry and kiwi salad with soy cream, Cream—mango sauce with soy milk and sunflower seeds, etc.

How to Deal with Depression

Depression is not uncommon. Moreover, in Western countries, it has become so common, that the name of the antidepressant, like, for example, of Prozac, right now, probably, on everyone's lips. The reasons for depression are many, but perhaps, you will be surprised, having learned that one of them may have a reaction to food.

Depression visits from time to time any of us, but we usually associate it with what—it is quite certain events. But many people suffer from depression, the causes of which are not at all obvious. Its degree ranges from mild depression to a constantly dejected state, and in extreme cases, people are generally not able to feel joy or even see no reason to live. Depression, as a rule, short-lived, and goes away, when life circumstances change for the better. But the rest of the states are alarming and require not only careful relationships but sometimes treatment.

Accepted food affects the processes, taking place in the brain. Some products cheer it up. Others are able to spoil it, suppress positive emotions. For some—the irony, the majority of products, improves mood, not very good for your health. As a result, when receiving them, as well as the rest, it is desirable to exercise restraint and caution.

Carbohydrates and Mood

When we eat foods containing carbohydrates and sugar, the brain receives more than tryptophan—an amino acid that improves mood. Tryptophan is found in protein products, but carbohydrates improve its absorption in the vessels of the brain. A lot of tryptophan is found in bananas, turkey meat, cottage cheese, and dried dates.

Nerve impulses are transferred between the nerve cells due to specific substances called neurotransmitters.

Depression Questionnaire

Use this questionnaire, to determine, if you are prone to depression.

1. Did you have trouble getting out of bed in the morning?
2. Are you having difficulty concentrating?
3. Have you recently suffered a bereavement, or have you broken your relationship with a loved one?
4. Do you not have the strength to deal with the case, which has always attracted you?
5. Have you lost your appetite?
6. Are you addicted to sweets?
7. Are you crying for no reason?
8. Do you live in the country, where there is little sunshine?
9. Do you feel that you have nothing to hope for, or is life meaningless?

If you answered "yes" to three or more of the questions, then you might be experiencing depression. Talk to your doctor and, in case, if you reveal depression, get help from him and from your dietitian.

Tryptophan is a precursor to serotonin, a neurotransmitter whose deficiency contributes to depression and depression. Antidepressants, such as Prozac, increase serotonin levels in the brain. This belongs to a group of antidepressant drugs, which are called selective inhibitors Reutilization Serotonin (SIRS). They inhibit the process of reusing serotonin in the brain, as a result of which it continues to be present, providing a good mood.

In the process of synthesis of serotonin is involved vitamin B 6. Include in your diet foods, rich in vitamin B 6; you agree to struggle with depression. Being in a depressed state, it is not without reason that we dream of enjoying sweets—ice cream, chocolate, or cake. Sweets affect the chemical processes in the brain. This is what, for example, occurs during dieting: you exclude from your diet foods rich in carbohydrates, which inevitably leads to the fact, that you develop a craving for it—when the desire to taste the sweet becomes obsessive, you break the diet.

Dopamine and Depression

With a lack of dopamine, you feel depressed; on the contrary, its increased amount improves mood. Although dopamine in the strict sense of the word is not a neurotransmitter, it also promotes the conduction of nerve impulses in the brain.

Dopamine is synthesized from tyrosine, one of the amino acids present in protein foods. Vitamin B 12 and B 9 (often referred to as folic acid), as well as magnesium are necessary for its formation. Among the products, rich tyrosine, are almonds, avocados, bananas, cottage cheese, lima beans, peanuts (raw, not salty), pumpkin, and sesame seeds. Vitamin B 12 lots in fish, dairy products, and spirulina.

- *Vitamins of group B Vitamin B 1 (thiamine)*
  Contained in brewer's yeast, brown rice, wheat germ, and soybeans.

- *Vitamin B 3 (Niacin or Niacinamide)*
  It is found in fish, eggs, brewer's yeast, cereal grains, and poultry.

- *Vitamin B 6*
  Contained in grains of millet, buckwheat, and oats, in crustaceans (shrimp, lobster) and in mussels.

- *Vitamin B 12 (cyanocobalamin)*
  Contained in fish and dairy products.

The Role of Zinc

There is a strong correlation between zinc and depression. We have often faced with patients, who are in a state of depression and who have found a lack of zinc. Postpartum depression is also associated with a lack of zinc, whose reserves are transferred from mother to fetus about a day before delivery. Zinc is necessary for the growth of the baby and for the development of its immune system. Restoring zinc in the mother's body after the baby is born helps prevent depression.

To verify whether there is enough zinc in your body, you can answer a short questionnaire on the right. If you decide to increase the zinc content, then follow, so that the amount does not exceed 50 mg per day, regardless of source (including—of multivitamin preparations). However, first, we advise you to consult a specialist—nutritionist.

Oysters, endive salad, alfalfa seedlings, seaweed, brown rice, asparagus, mushrooms, turkey meat, and radish contain a lot of zinc. Folic acid is found much in bovine liver, soya flour, green vegetables (especially— in broccoli), eggs, and brown rice. Sunflower seeds, green leafy vegetables, wheat germ, soybeans, mackerel, swordfish, and cod are rich in magnesium.

Check, if your body lacks zinc

Check how much you have zinc, answering the following questions.

1. Have you had white spots on the nails?
2. Do you rarely experience hunger?
3. Do you have pale skin?
4. Do you have stretch marks on the abdomen and back?
5. Do you have fat and, perhaps, acne-prone skin? Do you often catch a cold?

If you answered "yes" to two or more questions, you will, perhaps, not have enough zinc, and should be included in their daily menu foods, containing it. More precisely, check the level of zinc may be, examining its contents in sheared with neck thread. Almost all nutritionists can perform this simple and relatively inexpensive analysis for you.

Depression and Nutritional Deficiencies

There is a relationship between the number of certain vitamins (especially B vitamins) and depression. For people suffering from depression is characterized by low plasma levels, and many of them are mentioned, that diet-enriched food, rich in vitamins.

Group B has a beneficial effect on the symptoms. The most effective from the point of view of confronting depression are vitamin B 3, vitamin B 6, and zinc. Include in your daily menu rich in vitamin B 6 fish, and you will see how it will affect your mood.

Depression and Food Allergies

Many patients who come to us are asked to help them counteract depression. Often it turns out that the reason lies in the depression of food allergies or intolerances, and then deal with the problem is easier. And the symptoms appear in the form of dark circles under the eyes, skin diseases, insomnia, irritability, and feelings of anxiety.

"Guilty" foods can be determined using a simple blood test. However, in most cases, it is enough to simply remove one or more of the most likely allergens from the diet. Judging by our experience, this gives remarkable results.

The most common allergens in Europe are wheat, dairy products, and citrus fruits, while in the USA, corn is the dominant allergen. In addition, many "fast" meals, dyes, and food additives are considered allergenic. In rare cases, we have been allergic to celery or tomatoes.

The most notable example of the relationship with depression is allergies to gluten—people who develop celiac disease (cm.). If people suffering from this type of allergy do not avoid foods containing gluten, then the probability of depression in them will increase.

Useful Advice

Even our grandparents knew how useful every day to eat an apple— that truth is true to this day. Apples contain pectin, which helps remove lead from the digestive tract; This is especially important for those who live in cities with high pollution by exhaust gases.

Although many of our patients, who suffer from depression, achieved excellent results, excluding from your diet certain foods, such people, it is advisable to consult your doctor, especially if the depression is observed in them for a long time.

Tips for Combating Depression

When the blood circulates poorly, it reduces the level of oxygen and nutrients necessary for the brain—to overcome that you have to stand up and vigorously kneaded.

Improve blood circulation you can include in your diet foods, rich in antioxidants from the "magnificent five" (vitamins A, C, and E, and the minerals selenium and zinc), which are present in fresh fruits and vegetables, fish, and cereals. In addition, you need to add iron, necessary for the formation of red blood cells, which carry nutrients into the blood. A good source of iron is tripe (in particular, the liver), as well as apricots and raisins.

One of the factors contributing to depression, maybe the level of blood sugar (cm.). By consuming foods that promote an even release of carbohydrates throughout the day, you can avoid sudden spikes in your blood sugar. Eat more foods containing complex carbohydrates (whole grains and vegetables), in conjunction with a small amount of protein (meat, dairy products, nuts, and seeds). All this will allow you to maintain a balance of blood sugar throughout the day.

Are you enjoying this book? If so, I'd be really happy if you could leave a short review on Amazon, it means a lot to me! Thank you.

CHAPTER 5:

DISEASES AND MEANS FOR THEIR TREATMENT

Digestive System

Digestion is a complex physiological process, flowing almost non-stop, day and night, regardless of the fact, whether we work, train, or rest. But stress interferes with this process, slowing down or even completely interrupting it.

During the "fight or flight" reaction system, the digestive system is switched off, the energy flow is directed to where it is most needed— to defend, attack, or escape. Knowing this, we need to better understand what is subjected to stress our digestive system when we eat "on the run".

The digestive process is facilitated or inhibited, depending on the type of food consumed. Fruits, vegetables, whole grains, nuts, seeds, and proteins 1- grade (cm.) Improve digestion. Diet, rich in saturated fats, meat, sugar, caffeine, and fast food, slow digestion, is unsafe and reduces the absorption of essential nutrients.

Digestive Process

In order to understand what is happening in violation of digestion, you need to understand how the digestive system works. The digestive process begins from the moment when we are just starting to think about food or its scent. A signal is sent from the brain to the salivary glands, in response to which they secrete an additional portion of digestive enzymes. That is why, at the mere thought of appetizing food, we "salivate".

When chewing food, the digestive enzymes of the oral cavity quickly break down carbohydrates (fruits, vegetables, granola, cereals), turning them into gruel. Meat, nuts, and other proteins are more difficult to process; it requires an acidic environment and more powerful enzymes—those, that stand in the stomach. To properly process solid particles of food, it should be thoroughly chewed (more salivary enzymes are released), and the health and cleanliness of the teeth should be monitored. Most people don't give it due weight, and as a result, they expose their digestive system to increased stress, which often leads to heartburn and indigestion.

The stomach plays a key role in the digestion process. It is located behind the sternum and is protected on all sides by ribs. In all people, stomachs vary in shape and size. Observing the upright position during the meal, we provide the stomach with enough free space for the normal fulfillment of its functions. Hydrochloric acid is produced in the stomach, and the most acidic environment in the whole body is created inside it. (It also produces mucus in abundance, which protects the walls of the stomach from acid damage). Hydrochloric acid is involved in the breakdown of proteins, while the muscle walls of the stomach alternately contract and relax, contributing to the formation of food gruel.

The following factors can matter: old age, potent drugs, smoking, alcohol, stress, etc. when there is insufficient formation of acid developed numerous violations.

In addition, hydrochloric acid destroys bacteria and parasites. This is the first line of defense, built by the immune system, which lines the entire digestive tract. From the age of approximately 30 years, hydrochloric acid formation starts to decrease, which explains the increase in digestive system diseases and increases the frequency of food intolerance celebrated in old age.

However, the extremely aggressive Helicobacter pylori bacteria survive in the acidic environment of the stomach. In the absence of proper treatment with antibiotics, these bacteria can cause significant harm to the body.

Indigestion Symptoms

- Burping
- Food allergy
- Indigestion
- Itching in the anus
- Iron deficiency
- Nausea
- Bloating
- Headache
- Vitamin B 12 deficiency
- Cracked nails
- Worms
- Stomach upset
- Constipation
- Flatulence
- Acne

Chronic Candidiasis

The stomach also produces digestive enzymes. Pepsin contributes to the further processing of protein foods, facilitating the process of its digestion in the intestine. (For this purpose, vitamin B 6 is also necessary: eating sunflower seeds, ordinary beans, barley, broccoli, and cauliflower, we increase it content in the body). The process of digesting fats starts lipase.

In the final stage of gastric binding operation occurs external factor, vitamin B 12, with intrinsic factor, which is formed in the stomach, whereby the latter acquires the ability to be absorbed in the intestine. Vitamin B 12 plays a key role in the process of energy production, growth, and normal blood formation.

As they age, the level of internal factor decreases, which affects the absorption of vitamin B 12 and increases the possibility of pernicious anemia (vitamin B 12 deficiency).

That's why doctors sometimes prescribe injections of vitamin B to 12 sick, elderly people, and also recovering from surgery. Hydrochloric acid, in combination with digestive enzymes, contributes not only to better digestion of proteins but also to production of Vitamin B 12. In order to increase the level of this vitamin, eat more homemade cheese, haddock, halibut, tuna, and chicken.

Small Intestine

It is here that mainly digestion and absorption take place. Digestive enzymes that break down fats, proteins, and carbohydrates are secreted by the pancreas and contribute to the further processing of partially digested food slurry (chyme) in the stomach, preparing it for absorption in three sections of the small intestine: in the duodenum, jejunum, and ileum. The total length of these three sections is about 7 meters. However, all these intestines are compactly laid in the abdominal cavity.

The useful area of the small intestine is significantly increased by numerous tiny finger-shaped outgrowths on the inner surface, which are called villi. They secrete enzymes, absorb the necessary nutrients, and prevent food particles and potentially dangerous substances from entering the bloodstream. These sensitive processes can interfere with antibiotics and other medicines, alcohol, and/or excessive sugar intake. Upon contact with these substances, tiny gaps between the villi become inflamed and expand, as a result of which undesirable particles penetrate into the bloodstream. This is called increased intestinal permeability or "leaky gut" and can lead to food intolerance, headaches, fatigue, skin diseases, and arthritic pain in the bones and muscles of the whole body.

The duodenum is supplied bile, which is produced in the liver, and then concentrated and stored in the gallbladder. Bile is necessary for grinding particles of partially digested fats, as a result of which they acquire the ability to be absorbed. The pancreas secretes bicarbonate, which neutralizes or reduces gastric acidity, but also three secretes digestive enzyme protease, lipase, and amylase, required for digestion, respectively, of proteins, fats, and carbohydrates.

Useful Advice

To heal a stomach ulcer, drink a potato broth daily (boil the potato peel and strain the liquid) or potato juice (squeeze the juice from raw potatoes, and add carrot or celery juice for taste). Never pick potatoes with a green peel.

Skinny and ileum are the main base for the suction of the remaining nutrients, including protein, amino acids, water-soluble vitamins, cholesterol, and bile salts.

Ileocecal Valve

Between the small and large intestine has a tight valve, opening in one direction and intended for addition, to prevent a reverse flow of feces into the small intestine. This is the so-called ileocecal (iliac-cecum) valve, located very close to the appendix. In this area, inflammation often occurs, since bacteria and parasites can attach to the walls.

If inflammation is observed for a long time, the ileocecal valve may remain open, resulting in toxic substances penetrating the ileum with high absorption capacity. This can lead to an erroneous diagnosis of appendicitis and, as a result, to unjustified removal of the appendix, an important organ of lymphatic tissue. Therapy aimed at the destruction of parasites and bacteria, as well as a complete rejection of potentially irritating foods (grains, legumes, high in fiber) for a short time—all this allows you to heal the minor ailments without resorting to surgery.

Colon

The large intestine, or colon, consists of three consecutive sections (ascending, transverse, and descending colon), and ends with the rectum and anus. Colon active movements promote mixing of the contents (water, bacteria, insoluble fiber, and slag, formed after digestion of nutrients) and advancing it to the rectum and anus. The contents of the colon are removed through the anus in the form of feces.

Immediately after ingestion, the entire subsequent digestion process depends on the contraction of the musculature of the pharynx, and then on the esophagus, along which the food lump is advanced due to muscle contractions, like a crawling snake.

Feeling the desire to alleviate, it is advisable to go to the toilet and empty the intestines, because with a delay in feces, even for a couple of hours, further absorption of water occurs, and as a result, becomes drier, which contributes to constipation. This is also one of the causes of hemorrhoids.

"Normal" is considered to defecate at least once a day. In people with active digestion, the stool can be observed after each meal. On the other hand, stool retention can occur for several days—and then toxic substances again enter the bloodstream through the intestinal wall. That is why sometimes we experience a feeling of incomprehensible fatigue, headache, nausea, and general malaise. This explains the questions about the nature of our stool, which the doctor asks us at the reception for almost any reason.

Other problems, associated with the chair, discussed further.

Healthy Colon

To maintain the colon in perfect condition, you need to eat vegetables, fruits, and insoluble fiber, which is found in grains and legumes daily. In these products, magnesium is present which is necessary for the normal functioning of the intestinal muscles. If you can gather magnesium from vegetable or fruit juice, then in order to stock up on fiber, which helps to remove toxins from the gut and improve intestinal peristalsis, you should at least have a little fruit and whole vegetables.

For people who have undergone abdominal surgery, the postoperative period is necessary to very carefully monitor their diet because the departure of natural needs, they may be complicated for several days. It is advisable in the early days to take simple food that does not burden the intestines and reduces the likelihood of constipation. Vegetable soups, salads, steamed vegetables, and rice—all this is ideal for the postoperative period. These foods are rich in nutritionally, easy to digest, and contain enough fiber, to the rectum function recovered quickly.

Digestive Immune System

The digestive tract is 60-70% of the entire immune system of the body, and this is not surprising when you consider what a tremendous number of pathogens and potentially hazardous substances get into our body through the mouth—the gates of the digestive system. Billions of beneficial bacteria live in the oral cavity, esophagus, and small intestine, while there are trillions of them in the large intestine. But in the stomach, where the acidic environment reigns, there are not too many of them since there are few pathogenic microbes that can survive in such harsh conditions.

In total, from 400 to 500 species of various bacteria were found in the intestine, some of which have antitumor, while others, on the contrary, are carcinogenic; there are bacteria, which synthesize vitamins B, A and K; others produce substances that are opposed to certain infections; There are also bacteria that digest lactose (milk sugar) and regulate muscle contraction and relaxation. Intestinal bacteria secrete natural antibiotics and fungicides—substances that inhibit the growth of pathogenic bacteria and fungi, respectively. Highlighting acid, they also destroy the toxic products of harmful bacteria, which often pose a far more serious threat, than the actual disease-causing microbes.

In addition, the intestinal microflora protects us from metal poisoning—for example, mercury (from the amalgam present in seals or from infected fish), radionuclides (during antitumor therapy or from contaminated products), as well as pesticides and herbicides. There are also bacteria, which produce hydrogen peroxide, in the presence of cancerous cells die. However, as you'll see below, there are many factors, which disturb the normal balance of the intestinal microflora.

Beneficial bacteria should prevail in the gut in the absence of harmful factors, listed in the table (see below). If you eat poorly and monotonously, regularly consume alcohol, undergo stress, often use antacids, painkillers, and antibiotics, then the fragile balance will inevitably be upset. And then, the pathogenic bacteria will be able to multiply uncontrollably and displace the beneficial microflora.

Unfortunately, this way of life is inherent in quite a few. Such people suffer from indigestion, bloating, flatulence, and cannot understand what is the reason for their troubles. The answer is simple: their intestines have become a battlefield of beneficial and pathogenic bacteria.

Typical Lifestyle Factors That Negatively Affect Digestion

- Antibiotics
- Diet, rich in fats
- Sugar
- Refined Products
- Anti-inflammatory drugs
- Fried food
- Alcoholic drinks
- Canned drinks (carbonated)
- Stress
- Bereavement
- Smoking
- Stimulant drugs

Constipation

The main cause of constipation is dehydration. Constipation itself often causes headaches. To meet the needs of the body and to prevent constipation per day, you need to drink 1.5—2 liters of mineral still water. With strong physical exertion, this volume should be doubled. Constipation can occur from—the predominance in the diet of protein foods, with the failure of fiber, as well as high consumption of alcoholic beverages, tea, coffee, and other beverages containing caffeine—they all have a dehydrating effect.

To avoid constipation, you need to include in your diet a large amount of soluble fiber, which is found in vegetables and fruits, as well as insoluble fiber, which is found in rice, barley, buckwheat, and other cereal grains. (If you suffer from constipation, and do not drink enough fluids, then keep in mind: all legumes will only aggravate your problem, contributing to a thickening of feces).

Constipation is a fairly common occurrence during pregnancy, and it is often caused by iron supplements. Both of these problems can be solved if we take in food-soaked apricots overnight: in addition, that dried apricots contain a lot of iron, it is also a mild laxative. However, during pregnancy without consulting a doctor is entirely abandon the tablet, containing iron, it is not necessary.

Candidiasis

Candidiasis concerns many people. The causes of this disease are not entirely clear, but it is believed that his main culprits are improper diet and impaired immunity. Fungus Candida albicans is part of the normal intestinal microflora and behave innocently enough until there is a malfunction in the immune system, or if you have not switched to a diet which is rich in sugar. But then these fungi mutate into potentially dangerous microorganisms. The first signs of candidiasis are bloating, flatulence and intestinal colic after eating fruits and other sugary foods. In the absence of proper treatment, the condition is aggravated, and the patient feels constant fatigue and even depression. Less obvious symptoms of candidiasis include insomnia, ear itching, shoulder pain, irritability, inability to concentrate, sore throat and muscle pain, restless behavior, and acne.

One of the main causes of candidiasis is frequent antibiotic treatment. They, of course, are necessary for the fight against bacterial infection, but at the same time, destroy the beneficial intestinal microflora. In this case, there are conditions favorable for the reproduction of Candida albicans, which is often described as the growth of yeast.

Celiac Disease

Celiac disease, or gluten intolerance, is the disease in which the intestinal villi are flattened after exposure to gluten. Celiac disease can contribute to indigestion, diarrhea, weight loss, and general malaise. Condition is quite common and, perhaps, inherited. In infants, it usually manifests itself in the weeks after transfer to solid foods, gluten-free, but it can develop at any age.

People suffering from celiac disease cannot tolerate gluten in any form, so they should be excluded from the diet of the food wheat, barley, oats, and rye. In addition, doctors usually recommended in addition to gluten to abandon all starchy foods and grains, including rice and corn, as well as potatoes. In our opinion, this is not necessary. Many people suffering from celiac disease feel good if their diet includes plenty of fresh fruits, vegetables, fish, chicken, and grains, do not contain gluten.

Diverticulitis

In this disease sensitive membrane, lining the colon, inflamed, forming tiny sacs, or diverticula. Toxins get into these bags; inflammation intensifies, pain occurs. In complicated cases, surgery may be required.

Symptoms of diverticulitis include: diarrhea or constipation, soreness, bloating, and, most typically, frequent urges to empty the intestines. The development of diverticulitis is facilitated by constipation, to avoid which it is recommended to introduce more fiber and unsaturated fats into the diet, as well as drink more.

A therapeutic diet for diverticulitis, in addition to increasing fiber, class 1 proteins, and heavy drinking, is based on a decrease in carbohydrate intake (especially simple ones). Homemade vegetable soups excellent help during the attack, due to the abundance they contain nutrients, which are easily absorbed, without causing irritation to the intestines.

Diarrhea

Diarrhea is caused by various reasons, and often itself a symptom of some—any disease. Acute diarrhea is common with any infectious disease. Bloody diarrhea is a sign of acute inflammation—in such cases, it is necessary to consult a doctor.

Periodic diarrhea can be caused by food allergies, parasitic infections, pancreatic disease, caffeine abuse, and excessive stress.

With diarrhea, the body loses a lot of water and valuable minerals. Try to make up for the loss immediately after the attack with mineral-rich foods such as nuts, greens, and seaweed. Potassium loss should be compensated immediately—a lot of potassium is found in avocados, chard, lentils, parsnips, spinach, fresh nuts, sardines, and bananas.

If you occasionally have diarrhea, food may be the cause. Try to change the diet of their food, and, perhaps, things will go smoothly. Otherwise, consult with a specialist—a nutritionist or your doctor.

Food Poisoning

Food poisoning occurs after the absorption of any—or toxic substances, most often—pathogenic bacteria.

Symptoms of poisoning can occur within a few minutes after the ingestion of toxic food, although the activity of some types of bacteria may occur a week later. In the latter case, the patient is difficult to understand what caused the poisoning. It is likely. Therefore, food poisoning is more common than we are accustomed to thinking.

Bacteria, capable of causing food poisoning, a lot: it is Salmonella typhimurium, and Escherichia coli (E.coli), and the most dangerous Clostridium botulinum. Symptoms of food poisoning include chills, fever, chronic diarrhea, and muscle paralysis. In addition, nausea and vomiting may occur.

At the slightest suspicion of food poisoning, you should immediately consult a doctor. A good natural antidote is garlic, in addition, to compensate for the lost minerals. You should eat foods rich in potassium, for example, fruits and herbs. Living bio-yogurt will help you repopulate your intestines with beneficial bacteria. Activated charcoal in tablets sorb toxins well, so take it at the first sign of poisoning. To avoid poisoning, take all the precautions. At the slightest suspicion, that the food is poor quality, do not touch it!

In any case, taking a garlic pill before meals will help to neutralize pathogenic bacteria. If in the restaurant you can only hope for the honesty of the cooks, then at home you can take all measures to prevent poisoning. Use our tips.

Heartburn and Dyspepsia

With heartburn, caustic acid is expelled from the stomach into the esophagus, and a burning sensation and pain occur in the chest. With dyspepsia, the symptoms are similar, but pain is felt only in one place.

Usually, doctors recommend taking antacids to get rid of heartburn and dyspepsia, but this is a double-edged sword. The fact is that prolonged use of certain antacids can lead to a violation of the fine acid-base balance (pH) of the body. Buffer systems, used by the body to maintain its pH, cannot withstand the load, and combination with food, too rich in proteins, may cause damage to the kidneys.

Food Hygiene Basics

Wash your hands thoroughly before eating.

Warm food, or keep it in the cold; Avoid room temperature.

Please note that when cooked food is warmed up, it is done carefully and evenly.

If you eat meals in the open air, then move on to the food, as soon as the table is set. Do not leave food in the sun.

Do not buy canned goods in damaged or swollen cans, even if you are offered them for cheap. No savings will compensate you for the harm caused by possible food poisoning.

Catching up on cooking, watch out, the meat does not come into contact with other foods. Stock up on two to three chopping boards for different products. Wash hands thoroughly after handling raw meat.

We advise many patients whose condition is due to the consumed food. If you are prone to indigestion or heartburn, you need to eat easier. Having eaten a lot of protein, raw and fried foods in one sitting, you overload the digestive system. Eat should be slowly, chewing food thoroughly. Do not swallow anything scorching hot or supercooling. If the disorder is not to be held, talk to your dietitian—it will check whether it is related to food intolerance or enzymatic deficiency.

If your dyspepsia develops suddenly and does not go away, be sure to consult your doctor.

Hiatal Hernia

With a hiatal hernia, a part of the stomach is protruded into the chest cavity through the enlarged esophageal opening of the diaphragm as a result of which the gastric contents are thrown into the esophagus. Symptoms include belching, dyspepsia, belching and burning, caused by contact with acidic gastric juice by thin walls of the esophagus. Ultimately, this can lead to an esophageal ulcer.

As a therapeutic measure, it is useful to drink aloe infusion twice a day, which can be bought at any pharmacy. To alleviate bitterness, you can recommend a specially flavored infusion. For tissue regeneration, zinc is needed, a good source of which is pumpkin seeds, cereal grains, eggs, turkey meat, as well as oysters, lobsters, mussels, and crabs.

Hemorrhoids

With hemorrhoids, a pathological expansion of the veins occurs surrounding anus. The patient experiences pain, heaviness in the anus. Marked: swelling of the nodes, itching, burning, and hemorrhoidal bleeding. (Remember, that at the slightest sign of blood in the stool should immediately consult a doctor).

The development of hemorrhoids contributes to a diet with a lack of fiber and water; attempts at defecation lead to an additional load on the veins. To soften the stool and facilitate the excretion of feces, more greens, and whole grains and food containing fiber should be included in the diet. For the healing of cracks need food, rich in calcium and magnesium: vegetables, nuts, and seeds. Launched hemorrhoids require medical treatment.

Irritable Bowel Syndrome

According to the calculations of physicians, 15% of the UK population and 20% of the US population suffer sickness, known as irritable bowel syndrome (IBS). With IBS, normal peristalsis of the large intestine is disturbed, as a result of which toxins and waste products accumulate in it. In this case, patients note pain, bloating, diarrhea, and/or constipation. Often there is malabsorption.

Useful Advice

Blackcurrant has a fixing effect, and it is used to combat diarrhea. The canned berries vitamin C is much less than in fresh. Blackcurrant leaf tea is also useful.

To restore normal peristalsis, a complex of vitamins B is of great importance. They are rich in whole grains, fish, eggs, and wheat seedlings. To populate the intestinal beneficial bacteria necessary for the digestive tract and the synthesis of vitamins, it is desirable to take every day to eat a living bio yogurt. It is shown that patients with IBS required more proteins. There are many class 1 proteins in bean curd, fish, and chicken.

Apples promote the growth of beneficial bacteria in the large intestine. In addition, they contain pectin, which helps to remove excess cholesterol and toxic metals from the digestive tract.

Gastric and Duodenal Ulcer

With this unpleasant disease, ulceration of the mucous membrane of the stomach or duodenal wall occurs. Its main symptom is excruciating pain in the epigastric region, and as a rule, it gets worse after eating. In the occurrence of the disease, stress is given a large role, which violates the normal acidity of the stomach. Physicians are also advised to drink more water, to dilute the acidic juice and thereby reduce pain.

Avoid refined foods, salt, spicy seasonings, coffee, and fried foods—this also helps reduce pain and prevent further bouts. It is advisable to eat throughout the day more often, in small portions, and include whole grains, steam vegetables, and some class 1 proteins. Cabbage juice, which contains the amino acid methionine, which supports the liver's ability to neutralize toxic substances, is an effective treatment for ulcers. If you are over 30 and are tormented by acute pain, then you need to consult a doctor.

Helminthiasis

The human digestive system parasitizes many kinds of worms: the round (nematodes), flukes, and tapeworms. Worms parasitizing in the intestines can cause swelling, nausea, and general malaise. If you suspect carriage of worms, you should contact your doctor and consultant—nutritionist.

Crohn's Disease

Crohn's disease is characterized by inflammation and ulceration in the small and large intestines. Symptoms include weight loss, frequent severe diarrhea, persistent bloating, and food intolerance, which manifests itself in the form of chronic fatigue, muscle pain, various rashes on the skin. In acute cases, it may even involve surgical removal of part of the small intestine.

Dietary nutrition plays a very important role in this disease. To combat inflammation and excess mucus, wheat and dairy products must be completely abandoned. For products, aggravating the disease, also include citrus fruits, tomatoes, spicy foods, black pepper, coffee, cola drinks, and alcohol.

But the main thing in Crohn's disease is, to overcome the inflammatory process. During the first months, it is necessary to reduce the consumption of insoluble fiber: there are fewer fruits, especially strawberries and kiwi, which contain small grains that irritate the digestive tract. Healing especially includes a strict diet, including peeled potatoes, steamed fish, poultry, soft vegetables (e.g., zucchini, spinach), peas, and wild yam.

The main source of protein should be fish, which contains the well-known anti-inflammatory effects of vitamin E and omega- 3 polyunsaturated fatty acids. Both of these components are powerful antioxidants and have healing properties. The latter also applies to products, rich in zinc, e.g., meat, poultry, eggs, and seafood (they contain selenium, another antioxidant). But whole grains, also rich in zinc, should be excluded.

Ulcerative Colitis

It is a disease of the large intestine, which is characterized by bloody diarrhea, mucus in the stool, and acute pain.

Although patients require fiber, not every variety of fiber is suitable for this purpose. Like other nutritionists, we recommend limiting the intake of insoluble fiber (it is in the sweet corn and those rich in starch vegetables, like carrots, turnips, parsnips, and rutabaga) because digestion with this disease is difficult. Whole grains, nuts, and seeds should also be avoided. But boiled white rice, especially with garlic, has a beneficial effect on the digestive tract.

Simple carbohydrates and sugar—bread, biscuits, cakes, pastries, and pasta—should also be excluded from the diet. Wheat is irritating and can make the healing process difficult. Try to check the products if they contain wheat.

Sufferers from this disease noted that the state of their digestive tract is improved, if not to eat three times a day, and fractional and small portions. Dinner should be light. Desirably, to diet included more soluble fiber, which is contained in fruit and leaf green (and squeezed from it juices), for example, in parsley, watercress—salad, Kochan, and collard greens, spinach. Thanks to them, the body will receive the necessary fiber, which does not have an irritating effect on the intestinal wall.

Vitamin E is needed for the healing process, so we recommend eating more avocados, cabbage, and yams; they reduce inflammation and have antiulcer action. Anti-inflammatory activity is also characteristic of omega- 3 polyunsaturated fatty acids, which are rich in fatty fish: salmon, tuna, herring, sardines, and mackerel. Sunflower and pumpkin seeds are also useful. Try only to buy cold-pressed oils and do not heat them.

And Crohn's disease and ulcerative colitis are very serious diseases, threatening at times very dangerous complications. In addition to medical nutrition, do not forget to consult with your doctor.

Immune System

The immune system, perhaps, the most sophisticated and cleverly arranged system of our body. It almost always fights against potentially dangerous microorganisms that invade from the outside. It is likely that, at the same time, when you read this, your immune system is fighting desperately with a whole army of pathogens (microscopic harmful bacteria or viruses).

Pathogenic microorganisms are present everywhere—in the air, on the ground, in water, and in food products. Our body is also one of our favorite shelters for germs; innumerable hordes of them live on the skin, in the hair, under the nails. And yet—in our body. If the immune system does not cope with pathogens, then an infection develops.

How often do we remember about our immune system? Many people have heard that during colds useful to take dietary supplements, vitamin C, and drink plenty of orange juice, but their knowledge of these often limited. Although in order, to understand all the intricacies of immunological mechanisms, may not be enough and a few decades, a basic knowledge of immunology should, in our opinion, to learn each—only then will you understand how important for immunity have a proper diet and your lifestyle. But now you can learn how things do you do with the immune system, by replying to the questionnaire.

Basic Protection

Dodgy defensive systems, constructed by our body for protection against various troubles, we can only admire. The first line of defense is the skin, which is a natural barrier. Its surface is protected by the secretion of the sebaceous glands, which prevents the growth of some bacteria. Sweat glands located in the skin also contribute to the fight against potentially dangerous microorganisms—the released sweat removes microbes from the skin surface.

A similar protective function is also performed by the lacrimal ducts of the eyes, releasing fluid, which washes away the particles and eye irritants. In the summer, it is especially noticed the people suffering from hay fever—their eyes are always tearing of contact with the countless grains of pollen.

In the air, we inhale, the large number of harmful particles, which is fighting the respiratory tract. The internal airway epithelium is lined with tiny hairy outgrowths (cilia) that trap these particles. The trapping of foreign particles contributes to the mucous released here. The latter contains the so-called secretory immunoglobulins A (sIgA), which have the ability to neutralize pathogens.

Diseases and Their Treatment Questionnaire: Your Immune System

How effective is your immune system? To get an idea about this, answer the following questions.

1. Do you often have colds or flu?

2. If you have a cold, is it hard for you to get rid of a cold?

3. Do you often feel stressed?

4. Are you depressed or depressed?

5. Do you have a food allergy?

6. Do you regularly use painkillers?

7. Do you suffer from hay fever?

8. Over the past year, have you used antibiotics more than once?

9. Sore throat—not uncommon for you?

10. Do you drink alcohol more than three times a week?

11. Do you often have a headache?

If you answered "yes" to three questions, then, perhaps, you should pay more attention to your immune system.

If you answered "yes" to four questions, then your immune system is, obviously, needs closer attention.

Five or more positive answers indicate that your immune system cannot cope with the load.

The saliva in the mouth helps to get rid of bacteria, penetrate into the mouth air—droplets, or with food. After swallowing, saliva in the stomach mixes with gastric juice, which contains hydrochloric acid.

Most bacteria die under the influence of this acid, but such as Heli with obacter pylori, survive. If how—the micro-organisms can overcome the gastric barrier and get into the intestine, in the fight with them comes a useful local microflora.

Thus, our organism is protected from the outside and inside. Nevertheless, sometimes, despite all the efforts of the immune system, pathogenic microorganisms manage to cope with all the barriers, and then the disease occurs.

Immunological Armada

What happens, when we happen to swallow or breathe in harmful microbes? In these cases, the immunological host protects us in the same way as the flotilla to defend themselves against the enemy strategically important island—our body. The components of the naval forces not only prevent the invasion but also detects and eliminates all those who started behaving suspiciously in the ranks of the defenders—for example, cancer cells. Naval commanders keenly follow events and throw their ships there, where there is a need.

The fleet consists of immunocompetent cells. Some of them are floating around the body in search of the enemy, while others sit in ambush and attack the enemies, who are nearby. Wanderer cells are otherwise referred to as macrophages. In the process of phagocytosis, they swallow and digest pathogens.

Usually, immunocompetent cells are carried by blood. Distinguish between red and white blood cells (cells), which perform different functions.

Red Blood Cells

These cells, otherwise called erythrocytes, represent the most numerous categories. They are formed in the bone marrow, from which they enter the bloodstream. The main function of red blood cells is the transport of oxygen throughout the body, but, in addition, they have the ability to attract pathogens, followed by those, in turn, pay attention to the white cells. Red blood cells live very briefly and, having fulfilled their mission, are destroyed.

White Blood Cells

These cells, otherwise called leukocytes and lymphocytes, they are divided into several types, and their main function is protective. Some of them fight parasites and allergic reactions (for example, hay fever and asthma), while others counteract inflammation and infections.

An important variant of lymphocytes is helper T-cells. When a pathogen is detected, they instantly send a warning signal, tuning the immune system to repel an enemy attack. In the case of HIV-infection affects these cells, causing the immune system is disarmed.

CHAPTER 6:

AMAZING RECIPES

Rice Water

Preparation:

Boil in 1 liter of water 2 tablespoons of rice until the grain softens a lot and begins to disintegrate; then let it cool and strain it. Sweeten with a little sugar and aromatize with cinnamon sticks if you like.

Degreased Chicken Soil

Ingredients:

- 1/2 chicken
- 2 liters of water
- 1 large carrot
- 1/2 chopped onion
- 2 bay leaves
- 2 sprigs of fresh to-millo

Preparation:

1. In a pot, pour the water and chicken; bring to boil.
2. Add carrot, onion, bay leaves, and thyme; Let cook uncovered for 3 hours.
3. Remove the pot from the heat and strain the broth.
4. Cover it and put it in the fridge until the grease has solidified on the surface.
5. Remove the layer of grease and leave it in the fridge until you are going to use it.

Rice in the Oven with Merluza

Ingredients:

- 100 grams of rice
- 100 grams of hake
- water or broth
- virgin olive oil and salt

Preparation:

1. Put rice and a double measure of water or broth on the baking sheet.
2. Clean the hake and cut it into pieces.
3. Once the liquid has been poured, place the hake pieces on top.
4. Baking is exactly 18 minutes.
5. When it is taken out of the oven, it is left to rest 8 or 10 minutes before serving.
6. It is recommended that it be covered while it cooks and that it stays that way also when it comes out of the oven.

Cream of Zucchini

Ingredients:

- 2 medium zucchinis
- a portion of skimmed-salt and salt

Preparation:

1. First, peel and slice the kabobs, then put them in a pot to make them go through.
2. Remove them when they are tender, pass them by the blender, and then by the Chinese.
3. Pour the crushed in a saucepan along with the cheese. Stir until it is well bound.
4. Put salt to taste.

Thyme Soup

Ingredients:

- A good handful of thyme, preferably flowery
- 4 slices of white bread
- virgin olive oil,
- salt
- an egg (optional)
- 1/2 clove of garlic (optional)

Preparation:

1. Make a thyme tea with 1 liter of water.
2. Give a single boil (3 minutes over low heat).
3. Immediately, put the toasted bread on top and boil for 5 minutes.
4. Dress with a little oil and some chopped raw garlic.
5. Another option is to make a stir-fry with the garlic cut in slices, and when they are browned, add the toasted bread slices to absorb the stir-fry.
6. Add the thyme tea as explained above and boil for 5 to 10 minutes so that the bread is soft.
7. Put in the claypan and baked, putting the egg on top until it is cooked without the yolk fully set.

Cinnamon Membrillo

Ingredients:

- 2 quinces
- cinnamon sticks
- 1 tablespoon of sugar
- the skin of a lemon

Preparation:

1. Put in a pot the peeled and chopped quinces, the cinnamon stick, the sugar, and the lemon peel.
2. Add 2 glasses of water so that the quinces are covered and cover the pot.
3. Cook over low heat until the quinces are tender.
4. Serve them when they cool.

Apple Sauce

Ingredients:

- 1 kilo of sweet apples
- 1 glass of sugar
- 1 cinnamon stick
- 1 lemon

Preparation:

1. Peel the apples, then cut them into thin slices.
2. In a casserole, put apples with sugar, lemon peel, and a piece of cinnamon stick.
3. Pour water until the food is covered and bring to a boil.
4. Stir with a spoon so that the sugar dissolves and let it simmer for about 1 hour until the apple is soft.

Sweet of Membrillo

Ingredients:

- 1 kilo of quinces
- 1 kilo of sugar

Preparation:

1. Wash the quinces and cut them into quarters, removing the nuggets and hard parts.
2. In a pot cover the quinces with water, boil them until they are soft.
3. Strain the quinces and pass them through the blender and then through the small hole Chinese.
4. Put them on the fire again and add the sugar stirring with a spoon.
5. Remove them before the sugar burns.
6. Pour the contents into a mold and let it stand; it will take more consistency.

Sangría de Cítricos

Before lunch, you can have a juice, cocktail, or citrus sangria to whet your appetite.

Ingredients:

- 1 lime
- 1 lemon
- 1 orange
- 1 liter of white grape juice
- 1/2 of siphon
- crushed ice

Preparation:

1. Cut the lime, lemon, and orange in two.
2. Squeeze the juice one out of every two halves and cut the remaining into thin slices.
3. In a jar, mix grape juice, siphon and juice, and slices of lime, lemon, and orange.
4. Fill a glass with crushed ice up to 1/4 of its capacity, pour the sangria, and put a slice of fruit in each cup.

Oven Potatoes with Casted Cheese

Ingredients:

- 2 large potatoes
- 1/2 chopped onion
- 1 tablespoon of flour
- salt and pepper
- 1 glass of milk to which we can add a tablespoon of powdered milk
- 2 tablespoons of grated cheese

Preparation:

1. In a baking dish, form a layer with sliced potatoes.
2. Sprinkle with half the onion and then with half the flour.
3. Season with salt and pepper to taste.
4. Make another layer the same.
5. Pour hot milk on top.
6. Sprinkle with cheese.
7. Put the dish in the oven at 180C for 45 minutes or until the potatoes are tender.

Beans Cream

Ingredients:

- 50 grams of beans
- 1 glass of milk to which we can add a tablespoon of powdered milk
- a small bowl of béchamel sauce
- 1 teaspoon of butter
- salt and pepper

Preparation:

1. Soak the beans for several hours.
2. Boil them in saltwater.
3. When they are cooked, pass them through the blender.
4. Put the bean puree in a casserole together with the béchamel sauce.
5. Season with salt and pepper.
6. Add the milk and stir the mixture until you get the creamy consistency you want.
7. At the time of serving the mash, put the butter so that it melts.

Winter Salad

Ingredients:

- 1 turnip
- chopped escarole leaves
- 1 carrot
- 1/2 apple
- 2 tablespoons of raisins, nuts
- 1 natural yogurt enriched with cream
- 1 teaspoon of lemon juice

Preparation:

1. Grate the turnip, carrot, apple, and pontoon with the chopped escarole.
2. Mix everything with yogurt and lemon juice.
3. Grind the nuts and sprinkle them on top.

Broccoli with Bechamel

Ingredients:

- 1/2 kilo of broccoli
- 1 egg, butter
- milk
- virgin olive oil
- salt and pepper

Preparation:

1. Stripping broccoli from their fat trunks and outer leaves.
2. Put them in a steamer pot for 20 minutes.
3. Meanwhile, prepare a glass of béchamel, adding pepper at the end.
4. Cook the egg until it is very hard and peel it.
5. Oil a re-fractional source and place the broccoli, covering them with the béchamel.
6. Garnish with sliced egg and bake and gratin 5 minutes.

Spaghetti with Dry Fruits

Ingredients:

- 100 grams of spaghetti
- peeled walnuts
- 6 peeled hazelnuts
- 1 tablespoon of pine nuts
- 1 tablespoon of butter
- salt, virgin olive oil
- 1 tablespoon of grated Parmesan cheese
- Pepper
- 5 tablespoons of cream milk

Preparation:

1. Put salt and a tablespoon of oil in a tall pot with plenty of water.
2. When it is boiling, put the spaghetti for about 5 minutes until they are al dente.
3. In a mortar, crush the pine nuts, walnuts, and hazelnuts until the dried fruits are reduced to dust.
4. Mix them with 1 tablespoon of butter, about 5 tablespoons of cream of milk, and a pinch of pepper until you get a uniform paste.
5. When the spaghetti is al dente, drain them well and throw them in a bowl.
6. Add the nut paste, stir with wooden spoons, sprinkle the dish with grated cheese, and they are ready to serve.

Milk with Strawberries

Ingredients:

- 250 grams of strawberries
- 1 liter of milk
- 6 tablespoons of sugar
- 150 grams of cream

Preparation:

1. Crush the strawberries and pass them through the chi-no strainer.
2. Mix this mash with the very cold milk and add 4 tablespoons of sugar, stirring well until a smooth paste is left.
3. Pour it into the glasses and pour over cream, which you will have mixed with the 2 tablespoons of sugar before.

Juices Rich in Iron and Folic Acid

Ingredients:

- 1/2 beet
- 50 grams of kale
- 2 large carrots

Ingredients:

- 175 grams of strawberries
- 50 grams of blackberries
- 1 apple

More Energy Juices

Ingredients:

- 1 mango
- 1/2 pineapple
- a crushed banana with a fork
- 1/2 glass of milk or a natural yogurt
- 1 tablespoon of dried coconut
- 1/2 teaspoon of honey
- 1 teaspoon of germ wheat

Ingredients:

- 250 grams of strawberries
- 10 raspberries
- 3 apricots
- 1/2 glass of milk or yogurt
- 1/2 teaspoon of honey
- 1 teaspoon of wheat germ

Multimineral Reinforcement Juices

Ingredients:

- 1 red pepper
- 6 lettuce leaves
- 1 large carrot.

Ingredients:

- 3 tomatoes
- 1 bunch of parsley
- 1/2 turnip

Multivitaminal Reinforcement Juices

Ingredients:

- A small bunch of grapes
- 1 nectarine

Ingredients:

- 2 kiwis
- 1 pear
- 2 apricots

Boniate Cream

Ingredients:

- 1 sweet potato
- 1 egg yolk
- 1 teaspoon of honey
- a little milk

Preparation:

1. Steam the sweet potato, and when it is tender remove it and remove the skin.
2. Pass it through the blender with a little milk and the egg yolk.
3. Finally, add honey.

Pumpkin Cream with Salvia

Ingredients:

- 200 grams of pumpkin
- 1 tablespoon of Parmesan cheese or grated sheep cheese
- 4 leaves of sage
- 1/2 sprig of rosemary
- 1/2 garlic
- 1 tablespoon of virgin olive oil

Preparation:

1. Cut the squash into cubes and steam until tender.
2. Crush the aromatic herbs very thin and put them together with the garlic and the oil in a deep pan.
3. Let simmer a few minutes, then add the pumpkin, mix it well, crushing the pumpkin with a fork, and let it simmer for about 5 minutes.
4. Remove from heat and pass it through the blender.

Avocado Mayonnaise with Potatoes

Ingredients:

- 1 ripe avocado
- 1 medium potato
- Mayonnaise

Preparation:

1. Steam the potato without peeling for about 20 minutes (punch it with a knife to make sure it is tender).
2. When the potato cools, peel and chop it.
3. For the sauce, add to the mayonnaise the pulp of a ripe avocado and mix it well.
4. Pour the sauce over the chopped potato.

Potato Soufflé

Ingredients:

- 4 medium-sized potatoes
- 1/2 glass of milk
- 50 grams of butter
- 2 eggs and salt

Preparation:

1. Put the washed potatoes in cold water with salt.
2. Let them boil and cook.
3. Remove their skin and crush them.
4. Add the butter, milk, and salt.
5. Beat the mixture with a whisk and add the egg yolks one by one while still beating.
6. Then add the whipped whites to a very firm snow and mix everything carefully.
7. Grease a souffle fountain with butter.
8. Pour the mixture and put the dish in the oven. Let it brown.

Cheese Croquettes

Ingredients:

- 1/2 kilo of potatoes
- 25 grams of butter
- 125 grams of cheese
- 2 eggs
- Salt
- very fine breadcrumbs
- virgin olive oil

Preparation:

1. Cook unpeeled potatoes in salt water.
2. Once cooked, peel and crush them with a fork until you get a very fine puree.
3. Grate the cheese and add it to the mashed potatoes, as well as the melted butter.
4. Mix it all well.
5. Separate the yolk from the egg white and incorporate it into the dough it has in the casserole, mixing it well.
6. When the paste is homogeneous, throw the clear that has previously beaten to the point of snow.
7. Use everything carefully.
8. On a plate beat the remaining egg and in another place the breadcrumbs.
9. With the pasta we have in the casserole, croquettes are formed, dipped in the beaten egg, and coated with breadcrumbs.
10. They are fried in hot oil. Let the croquettes cool before eating them.

Vanilla Ice Cream

Ingredients:

- 350 mL of milk
- 1 vanilla branch
- 100 grams of honey
- 2 egg yolks
- 200 grams of whipped cream

Preparation:

1. Pour the milk in a small saucepan.
2. Core vanilla throughout. Take out the seeds and pour the branch and the seeds into the milk.
3. Beat the honey and egg yolks in a bowl until the dough turns yellow and makes threads.
4. When it rises, remove from heat.
5. Separate the vanilla branch and slowly pour the milk into the egg yolk, stirring quickly.
6. Pour everything back into the saucepan and let it heat to a boil.
7. Add the whipped cream and then let the dough cool in a cold-water bath.
8. Pour the prepared dough into a metal container that has been previously frozen and put it in the freezer.
9. Stir thoroughly once every hour at the beginning, and then more often.

CONCLUSION

Thank you for making it through to the end of *Acid Reflux Diet*, let's hope it was informative and able to provide you with all of the tools you need to achieve your goals whatever they may be.

The recommendations in this book will be sufficient to control the condition in that patient who suffers from acid reflux in a more acute state, in the event that it is in a moderate or severe state, it should be complemented with medical treatment.

Avoid those factors that increase intra-abdominal pressure. In the event that you are overweight or obese, you will have to lose weight.

- Divide the diet into 4-6 doses, with low volume meals.
- Eat slowly, chew food well, and calmly. Avoid flatulent and fried foods.
- Avoid eating 3-4 hours before bedtime.
- Prioritize soft cooking such as oven, stew, microwave, or steam.
- Avoid extreme temperatures of food and beverages.
- Prevent the texture of food from being very liquid since it hinders the digestion process.
- Avoid copious and fatty foods.
- Avoid acidic and spicy foods when there is inflammation.
- Avoid smoking and drinking alcoholic beverages.
- Avoid foods and drinks that contain caffeine.
- Avoid drugs that can cause reflux.

Finally, if you found this book useful in any way, a review on Amazon is always appreciated!

CPSIA information can be obtained
at www.ICGtesting.com
Printed in the USA
FSHW021258130421
80444FS

9 781801 235853